NURSES' AIDS SERIES

Nurses' Aids Series

CARING FOR WOMEN
OBSTETRIC AND GYNAECOLOGICAL NURSING

4th Edition

Ruth Bevis RGN, RM, HV Cert, ADM
Part-time Practice Nurse in West London;
Formerly Midwifery Sister, Bristol Maternity Hospital

Baillière Tindall
London Philadelphia Toronto Sydney Tokyo

Baillière Tindall 24–28 Oval Road,
W. B. Saunders London NW1 7DX

The Curtis Center, Independence Square West
Philadelphia, PA 19106–3399, USA

55, Horner Avenue
Toronto, Ontario M8Z 4X6 Canada

Harcourt Brace Jovanovich (Australia) Pty Ltd.,
32–52 Smidmore Street, Marrickville, NSW 2204,
Australia

Harcourt Brace Jovanovich (Japan) Inc.,
Ichibancho Central Building, 22–1 Ichibancho,
Chiyoda-ku, Tokyo 102, Japan

© 1991 Baillière Tindall

First published 1969
Second edition 1975
Third edition 1983
Fourth edition 1991

A catalogue record for this book is
available from the British Library

ISBN 0-7020-1453-2

Typeset by Best-set Typesetter Ltd., Hong Kong
Printed in England by Clays Ltd, St Ives plc

CONTENTS

PREFACE

This new edition of the Nurses' Aids Series Obstetrics and Gynaecology, now entitled 'Caring for Women', has been written to try and keep abreast of the rapid developments taking place in these specialties. The aim has been to consider the care of the whole woman, so related subjects such as mastectomy and urinary tract problems have been discussed.

The obstetrics and gynaecology merge and overlap in places, although the author has tried to present all the material clearly in a logical sequence, so that the student may readily locate the information she or he requires.

The concept of care of the whole person is presented together with the recognition of individual needs. The nursing process provides a framework for this approach.

The subjects contained in the United Kingdom Central Council (UKCC) syllabus for the obstetric and gynaecology modules in the Registered General Nurse course are covered and further reading is suggested at the end of each chapter for more detail. This book is also relevant to student nurses on the adult general branch of Project 2000.

The role of the midwife has been discussed at some length in the first chapter, in order to give the student an understanding of how the practice of the midwife differs from that of the qualified nurse. After this the role of the midwife may not be mentioned frequently, but its importance is recognized throughout in the care of mothers and babies.

The author also recognizes the importance of seeing the care of mother and baby together. In the interests of clarity their care has been discussed in separate chapters, but this does not indicate any desire to see them as separate entities. The father too is not forgotten, and it is recognized that many men now want to be much more involved in all aspects of pregnancy and baby care. This is welcomed, though his presence may be assumed rather than mentioned in parts of the text.

One small but significant innovation is to refer to the pregnant woman as a 'woman' or a 'mother' rather than a 'patient', except where she is obviously ill and in need of nursing care. Women themselves want to move away from the 'medical model' in obstetrics, and those of us caring for them have begun to make moves in this direction. Obviously there will always be a medical aspect to obstetrics, and this is right and proper, but at the same time the professionals are becoming more relaxed, flexible, and less traditional in their approach to care. The consumers, aided by the media, have probably done more to change attitudes and methods of care in obstetrics than in any other field of medicine.

The student nurse will therefore find obstetrics very different, because the women and their babies are generally fit and healthy, and do not require their nursing skills in quite the usual way.

The author has tried to be sensitive to the student nurses as real people too, and has tried to air some of their difficulties in these demanding areas of caring. However, in a textbook of this size, this cannot be done in great detail, and so there is suggested further reading at the end of each chapter.

New features include a glossary and a list of useful addresses.

ACKNOWLEDGEMENTS

My thanks are due to Shirley Gibbs for her help with matters relating to contraception; also to Sue Snoxall and Una Stevens in the teaching department at Queen Charlotte's Hospital for Women, who kindly helped with the gynaecology chapters.

The gynaecological chapters were written in association with Margaret Rutter, RGN, SCM, OND, RNCT, RNT, Dip N (Lond) Dip NEd (Lond), ENB 901 (Family Planning Nursing Certificate), Nurse Tutor for Continuing Education, Gloucestershire College of Nursing and Midwifery, Cheltenham.

The chapter on the breast was written in association with Betty Kershaw, RGN, RNT, MSc (Nursing) Principal, Stockport, Tameside and Glossop College of Nursing, Ashton-under-Lyne.

Introduction

1

CARING FOR WOMEN

Women are different. No-one is likely to argue with that statement, neither the woman, who feels she is different, nor the man who endeavours to understand her, whatever his relationship to her may be. The 'differentness' of women stems from their sexuality and their reproductive capacity, both of which are influenced profoundly by psychological, emotional, cultural and hormonal factors.

The student nurse, in both obstetrics and gynaecology, is seeing women at all stages of their reproductive life, and in a wide variety of conditions. Some are desperate to become pregnant and cannot, some are pregnant and desperate not to be so; still others have had gynaecological surgery which has altered their whole body image and often, for a time at least, shaken their self-confidence. Even the woman who has intentionally had a baby has enormous physiological and emotional adjustments to make, as well as finding that her social standing and all her personal and family relationships have subtly shifted. Women's moral and religious beliefs will be as varied as those of the nurses caring for them and will colour their attitudes and life-style. All must be equally respected. Caring for women in obstetrics and gynaecology is a demanding specialty. The male nurse may find it a bewildering challenge.

THE NURSE AND HIS OR HER FEELINGS

Not only does the nurse have to care for women who may be emotionally labile and in need of patient understanding, but she has to face up to her own, perhaps unexpected reactions, which may be very strong. There are many emotive situations to encounter, and many moral and ethical dilemmas to consider. (A nurse who feels she cannot take any part in termination of pregnancy, for example, is of course at liberty to discuss this with senior colleagues, and to register her objections of conscience.)

CULTURE AND BACKGROUND

Cultural influences provide a fascinating study. For the girl who has grown up and left school with the single clear objective of becoming a wife and mother, in many cases without any intervening employment experience, life is perhaps relatively uncomplicated, though many of these girls later regret their early domestic ties and lack of financial freedom. The 'career woman', however, often decides in her thirties that total fulfilment has somehow passed her by, and that she desperately wants a baby. The urge to have a baby is a deep one (whether or not purely biological is an interesting debate), but Western society in the early 1990s still implies that being a full-time mother is somehow a second class occupation which atrophies the brain, and is rather mundane. While many women have the self-confidence to ignore these pressures and remain full-time mothers when their children are small, for others this may be a source of conflict. For financial reasons women may opt or be forced to work outside their homes while bringing up a family. The nuclear family is a much less well-defined and stable unit in the 1990s, and many parents are bringing up their children single-handed for a variety of reasons, and many families are extended to include step-children. Another important change which has taken place since the 1950s is that families have become much more mobile and grandparents have become less significant figures in child-rearing for many families. This means that mothers of young children, whether or not they work, do not receive as much day-to-day support as mothers of a previous generation might have done.

For women from immigrant communities life may go on much as it would in their own countries. Many such women may be isolated and protected from Western culture; they often speak very little English and their menfolk deal with many of the practicalities of daily life.

When communication is a problem interpreters should be used; most hospitals now have lists of individuals who are willing to help in this way. Women will sometimes have their husband or their child with them to translate and there may be a problem with accuracy or completeness of information relayed in either direction. For example, a husband may not wish to tell his wife that she is being advised not to have sexual intercourse for a period of time.

For second and third generation immigrants, westernized to a great extent by school life and the media, there may be tremendous pressures and conflicts on reaching maturity. Girls in their late teens may be firmly deflected from their career prospects and ambitions, and steered into arranged or semi-arranged marriages, followed often by a close succession of pregnancies. Resistance to such pressures may be extremely difficult.

WOMEN'S SEXUALITY

Another important factor for the nurse to consider is that not all the women she meets will be involved in a long-standing relationship, and that some women's sexual partners will be women. It is very important to question the patient sensitively, and in a carefully worded way. This is a situation which demands tact and understanding; the nurse must maintain a professional approach and refrain from voicing her own feelings and beliefs unless discussion is invited.

As well as being aware of all the factors influencing women's attitudes to their sexuality and fertility, the nurse needs to remember the intimate nature of the woman's condition, whatever it may be. In presenting herself to an obstetrician/gynaecologist, the woman subjects herself to questions of an intensely personal nature regarding her sexual activity, past and present, as well as to physical examination of an intensely personal nature, from a total or relative stranger. The nurse needs to bear in mind how acutely embarrassed the woman before her may feel, and to do all she can to allay the woman's apprehension, and to maintain her dignity.

SEXUAL VIOLENCE

The problem of sexual abuse is emerging much more than in the past. The woman who has been the victim of sexual violence—rape or other forms of abuse or assault—may have deep psychological problems and will need sensitive care and perhaps long-term counselling, whether the sexual violence was recent or in the past. She may have difficulty accepting the need for vaginal examination, particularly by a male doctor.

WOMEN AND HEALTH

Women tend to be much more aware of health issues in the early 1990s. The contents of supermarket trolley have changed considerably in 10 years as women take more responsibility for their own healthy diets and those of their families. Self-help in health care is encouraged and advice and information on healthy life-styles is readily available to the more articulate sections of the population. Sadly, however, those who most need to be reached with health education remain the most ignorant, and the least receptive to advice. Despite efforts in schools, youth clubs and the media, young people continue to be sexually active and in some cases promiscuous from a young age, to smoke and abuse drugs and solvents. Cervical screening is available to all women who are sexually active, as is free contraceptive advice and prescribing (with the odd exception of condoms in some situations). Women are encouraged to examine their own breasts regularly and in some areas mammography is becoming more readily available as a screening measure. Health screening for women is discussed in more detail in Chapter 33.

Many women seek self-help in alternative medicine, and find relief for stress symptoms, premenstrual syndrome and problems associated with the menopause. Health food shops usually stock homeopathic remedies. With all the pressures on NHS resources and more recognition of the value of the holistic approach, alternative therapies such as osteopathy, acupuncture, homeopathy and aromatherapy are now seen as more 'respectable' and less on the fringe of medical practice. As health educators, often in a very effective position, nurses should endeavour to be well informed about such sources of help as well as giving general health education whenever opportunity arises.

THE STUDENT NURSE AND OBSTETRICS

For the student nurse in obstetrics, an understanding of the team effort involved is very important. The team may consist of the general practitioner and the midwife alone, or it may extend to include many other professionals. At the other end of the spectrum, in a busy consultant unit, the pregnant or newly delivered mother may meet radiographers, physiotherapists, dieticians, the paediatrician and the anaesthetist, as well as the obstetrician and the midwife. The nursing team will also be very varied. Finally the new mother and baby return to the primary health care team, with the midwife, general practitioner and the health visitor.

CHANGES AND PROGRESS

At the turn of the century, death and disease or damage were still rampant among newly delivered mothers and their babies. The team effort we see today is aimed at reducing maternal and infant mortality and morbidity. Statistics have improved tremendously since the early 1900s, but the figures are still too high. Since the inception of the National Health Service (NHS) in 1948 we have moved in the United Kingdom to being able to offer every pregnant woman a hospital confinement and much higher standards of care. The reaction of many has been to feel that the vastness of the 'system' depersonalizes women, and that medical intervention has been excessive. The vocal minority of women has made itself heard and many women wish, quite rightly, to have some control over what happens to them in pregnancy and labour. Those involved in the care of mothers and babies have therefore had to stand back and take careful stock of all they are doing. There may be conflict, apparent or real, between the ideals of the obstetrician and the wishes of the woman and her partner in some circumstances. The diplomat who has to please both parties and to encourage them to cease hostilities, if the situation has reached that point, is the midwife.

The World Health Organization says of the midwife:

> The midwife is a practitioner in her own right, with certain statutory responsibilities, who is trained to care for the mother and baby before, during and after delivery. She is expected to detect any abnormality at any stage and to refer these to the appropriate person.

Midwives are emerging from a period of uncertainty when they were fearful of greater medical involvement and the technological advances of the 1970s, and are recognizing their continued importance alongside recent advances. A close relationship can develop between mother and midwife (and frequently father too) and if it can start in the antenatal period and continue right through until mother and baby start seeing their health visitor regularly, so much the better. This is an ideal often not realized and so midwives have the challenge of meeting women at an intensely personal and important event in their lives, and of developing a good relationship in a very short time.

It has already been suggested that the ideals of the obstetrician and the wishes of the couple may not appear entirely compatible. Some women are anxious not to be 'tied to the bed' with fetal monitoring equipment restricting movement. They wish to be ambulant throughout labour, have minimal and preferably no medical intervention, and to deliver in one of the 'alternative birth' positions, whichever they find the most comfortable at the time. Midwives must therefore be flexible, in more ways than one, since some alternative positions necessitate his or her taking up a less than dignified pose in order to assist the delivery. This whole approach to pregnancy and delivery, where everything is natural, is usually referred to as 'active birth', not to be confused with 'active management of labour', which is how the obstetricians describe what they do.

The team effort has also been mentioned, and this has been discussed from the point of view of the various professionals involved. However, the mother is increasingly involved in her own care, just as, whenever possible, the sick patient is involved in planning his or her individual care as the nursing process is carried out. Some couples want this, while others are not ready or willing to make the decisions regarding their care before, during and after labour. The caring team must be careful not to push responsibility for decisions onto people who do not wish to take it.

FURTHER READING

DONNISON, J. (1977) *Midwives and Medical Men*. London: Heinemann Educational.

GOULD, D. (1990) *Nursing Care of Women*. Englewood Cliffs, NJ: Prentice Hall.

KITZINGER, S. (1980) *Sheila Kitzinger's Birth Book*. London Fontana.

LEWIS, J. (1980) *The Politics of Motherhood*. London: Croom Helm.

MCPHERSON, A. & ANDERSON, A. (Eds.) (1983) *Women's Problems in General Practice*. Oxford University Press.

OAKLEY, A. (1979) *Becoming a Mother*. Oxford: Martin Robertson.

PRINCE, J. & ADAMS, M. (1978) *Minds, Mothers and Midwives*. Edinburgh: Churchill Livingstone.

WEBB, C. (1985) *Sexuality, Nursing and Health*. Chichester: Wiley.

WEBB, C. (Ed.) (1986) *Midwifery and Gynaecological Nursing* (Using Nursing Models Series). Sevenoaks: Hodder and Stoughton.

2

ANATOMY AND PHYSIOLOGY

THE FEMALE REPRODUCTIVE TRACT

Position

The female reproductive tract is situated deep in the pelvic cavity, protected by the bony cage of the pelvic girdle (Fig. 2.1). It is a small, symmetrical system equipped to facilitate the uniting of ovum and sperm, nurture the fertilized ovum throughout its development, until the time comes for its final role of expelling the new, unique individual.

Components of the system

Ovaries   These bilateral organs are concerned with the production and liberation of the egg cells (oocytes).

Fallopian tubes   These bilateral hollow tubes are designed to transport the discharged oocyte to the uterus.

Uterus   This is a hollow, muscular organ, designed to protect and house the developing embryo (Fig. 2.2).

Vagina   This is the tube-shaped passage linking the internal and external genitalia.

Vulva   This is the external entrance to the system.

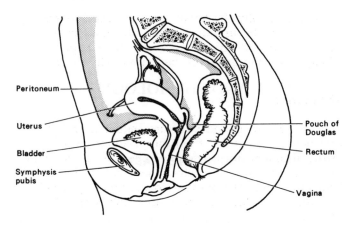

Fig. 2.1 Sagittal section of the pelvic organs.

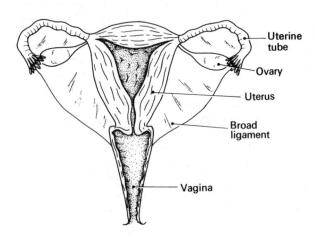

Fig. 2.2 The uterus and its appendages.

Embryologically the female genital tract develops in tandem with the urinary system, and this sometimes leads to anomalies of development (see Chapter 24— 'Congenital abnormality of the Reproductive Tract').

The ovaries

The ovaries are paired structures situated within the true pelvis, suspended from the posterior layer of the broad ligament by a double layer of peritoneum. The ovarian ligament, which lies within the broad ligament, connects the ovary to the uterus just below the junction of the fallopian tube (oviduct) with the uterus.

The ovary is the female counterpart of the testis, and its appearance and size varies according to age and the stage of the reproductive cycle. Females are born with ovaries containing thousands of specialized cells— oocytes—each of which has the potential to develop into a mature egg or ovum. At birth the ovaries are large compared to the uterus and their surface is smooth. By puberty the uterus has grown rapidly, and the ovaries have descended into the true pelvis. As the reproductive period of life progresses the ovary becomes increasingly scarred and uneven due to monthly eruptions of ripened follicles. In the normal non-pregnant female the rhythmic cycle recurs, the changes occurring in the ovary constituting the ovarian cycle, brought into play by the hormonal or pituitary cycle, and in its turn influencing a series of changes in the uterus, called the menstrual cycle (Fig. 2.3).

The fallopian tubes

These are thin muscular tubes, little bigger than an appendix, attached to the uterine body at one end, and opening freely into the peritoneum at the other, their

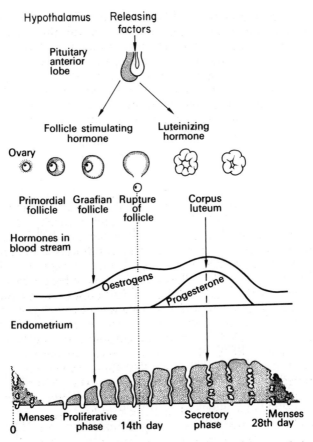

Fig. 2.3 **Diagram showing the hormones which influence ovulation and the menstrual cycle.**

trumpet-like ends fringed with fimbriated processes embracing the ovaries, ready to waft the oocyte into the adjacent lumen.

The tube provides the site for the uniting of the ovum (matured oocyte) and the sperm, which arrive there by the impetus of their own motility. The movement and peristalsis of the tube varies with the stage of the cycle, being more active at ovulation, when it is necessary for the tube to intercept the 'free fall' of the oocyte, and guide it into the entrance. The oocyte undergoes a final maturation to become an ovum capable of being penetrated by one sperm only. The fertilized ovum reaches the uterus approximately three to five days later.

The uterus

The uterus is a hollow, pear-shaped organ situated in the midline of the bony pelvis, and is ideally suited to the survival of the embryo. It provides a constant temperature, perfect metabolic conditions and protection from shock and injury. It has a unique muscle arrangement which allows an organ little bigger than a woman's fist, and weighing a few ounces, to expand and thicken to support and sustain a fetus weighing on average 3.5 to 4.5 kg at term. The main part of the uterus is called the body or corpus, and encloses a triangular cavity, the walls of which are normally in contact with each other, so that the uterine cavity is a potential rather than an actual space. The plain muscle fibres are in three layers, an outer longitudinal and inner circular one with a thick middle layer arranged in a criss-cross fashion and containing many blood vessels. The lining of the cavity is composed of columnar epithelium, the endometrium.

The cervix, or neck of the uterus, is cylindrical in shape and communicates with the cavity above by the internal os, and with the vagina below by the external os.

The muscle of the cervix is continuous with that of the corpus of the uterus (Fig. 2.4). The lining of the upper two-thirds of the cervix is columnar epithelium

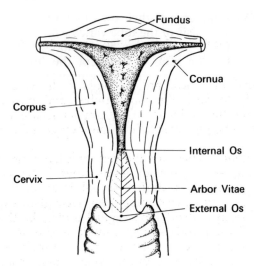

Fig. 2.4 Divisions of the uterus.

as in the uterus, but there is an abrupt change at the external os to the squamous type of epithelium. It is this site, referred to as the squamocolumnar junction, which is vulnerable to the development of carcinoma (see Chapter 29).

The vagina

The vagina is a muscular canal, lined with stratified squamous epithelium (skin), which is kept moist by the secretions of the uterine and cervical glands. The walls contain elastic as well as muscular tissue, which allows considerable stretching to take place during childbirth. The cervix projects into the upper part of the vagina, which is at right angles to the anteverted uterus (its normal position).

The vulva

The vulva consists of two bilateral folds of skin, the labia majora and minora.

Labia majora These are the outer folds which fuse anteriorly to form the mons pubis, and posteriorly merge into the perineum. They contain sebaceous and sweat glands, plus hair follicles on their lateral aspect.

Labia minora These are the very sensitive inner folds containing some erectile tissue around the clitoris providing sensation during sexual intercourse. The labia minora contain sebaceous and sweat glands which lie posteriorly, close to the vaginal orifice, Bartholin's glands. These glands secrete a lubricant during sexual excitement, and release it via a duct. Bartholin's duct is prone to blockage by thickened secretion or inflammation (Fig. 2.5).

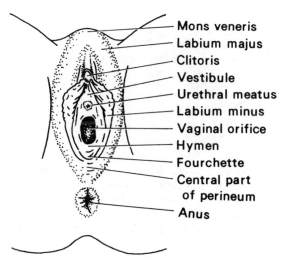

Fig. 2.5 The external genitalia.

THE PELVIC FLOOR

Sagittal section of the female pelvis shows the uterus in its normal anteverted position with the bladder nestling below and in front of it, and the upper rectum behind (see Fig. 2.1). The proximity of these structures and the angle of the uterus serves to prevent the sliding down of these structures, since there is no suspension from above. There is, however, support from below, necessary because of our erect posture, in the form of muscles and ligaments, in an area of soft tissue, shaped like a hammock, called the pelvic floor.

Muscles of the pelvic floor (Figs. 2.6 and 2.7)

Levator ani muscles   These are strong sheets of muscle arising from either side of the true pelvis, converging

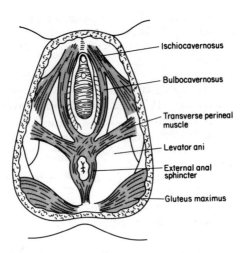

Fig. 2.6   The perineal muscles.

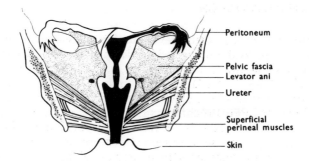

Fig. 2.7 The layers of the pelvic floor.

downwards and inwards to insertions at the central perineum, the anal canal, sacrum and coccyx.

These muscles support the pelvic and abdominal viscera, including the bladder. The muscle is pierced by the rectum, the vagina and the urethra.

The perineal body This is a pyramidal mass of fibro-muscular tissue which lies between the lower third of the vagina and the anal canal. It gives attachment to eight muscles:

Sphincter ani—this keeps the anus closed.
Bulbospongiosus—this muscle contracts the vaginal orifice during coitus.
Transverse perineal muscles (superficial)—a pair of relatively weak muscles, maintaining the position of the perineal body.
Transverse perineal muscles (deep)—a strong pair of deep muscles.
Levator ani—the anterior fibres of this pair of muscles are inserted into the perineal body.

The interlacing of these muscles with the fascia of the perineal body form a supporting sling and sphincter for the vagina, and so indirectly support the uterus and bladder. Any damage to these structures during childbirth may cause the vagina and even the uterus to subside through the pelvic floor; this is known as prolapse.

THE PELVIC PERITONEUM

The broad ligament

The body of the uterus is completely covered with peritoneum except for a narrow area extending laterally on each side, to form the broad ligament—a misnomer, since it is not a true ligament. The broad ligament contains the fallopian tube, the round and ovarian ligaments, and in its base, the ureter.

The pouch of Douglas

At the back of the uterus the folds of the peritoneum cover the posterior aspects of the cervix and upper vagina, reflecting back over the upper rectum to form a loop of peritoneum called the pouch of Douglas. The pouch of Douglas is important from a gynaecological point of view, as pus or blood may pool there following an abscess or tubal rupture.

The uterovesical pouch

Anteriorly the peritoneum covers the uterus to the level of the internal os, where it is reflected over the bladder, thus forming the uterovesical pouch. The peritoneum is loose here, as the bladder is an organ which needs to expand, fill and empty at intervals.

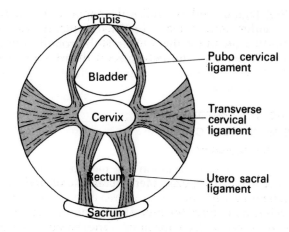

Fig. 2.8 The uterine supports seen from above.

Ligaments of the uterus

Pubocervical ligament Although more a fascia than a ligament, this structure passes downwards and forwards from the cervix to the posterior bodies of the pubic bone. It provides support for the bladder which rests upon it (Fig. 2.8).

Transverse cervical ligaments (cardinal ligaments) These ligaments, sometimes referred to as 'butterfly' ligaments, pass from the uterus and vagina to a wide insertion in the lateral pelvic wall, giving a fan-wise spread, which helps retain the uterus within the pelvis.

Uterosacral ligaments These ligaments help the round ligament to maintain the anteverted position of the uterus. They pass upwards and backwards from the cervix and vaginal vault to blend with the fascia of the sacrum.

Round ligament   Near the junction of each fallopian tube with the uterus is a cord-like structure encased within the broad ligament. This is the round ligament which keeps the uterus angled forwards. It passes through the inguinal canal and its fibres disperse in the labia majora.

THE MENSTRUAL CYCLE

The physical manifestation of menstruation is discussed in Chapter 22—'Menstruation and Associated Problems'.

The physiological events of the monthly cycle are controlled by the hypothalamus through the hormones of the anterior pituitary gland and the ovaries. Changes occur which affect the whole body.

The hypothalamus controls the autonomic nervous system and as such plays an important part in the stability of the body's internal environment. It also controls sexual function and reproduction.

The pituitary is subservient to the hypothalamus, its anterior lobe producing trophic hormones, that is, hormones which work by controlling other endocrine glands, in this case the sex organs or gonads. Under hypothalamic influence the pituitary produces two gonadotrophic hormones:

FSH: follicle stimulating hormone.
LH: luteinizing hormone.

Follicular phase

The follicular phase is characterized by the growth, maturation and rupture of an ovarian follicle (an oocyte enclosed in a secretory cavity). Immediately following menstruation the next cycle begins with the pituitary producing follicle stimulating hormone which leads to the development of several follicles in each ovary. The follicles go through various stages of maturation in response to FSH, but only one stays the course to full ripeness, by which time it has become a cystic, fluid-filled structure, known as a graafian follicle.

The graafian follicle

The graafian follicle, encircled by a supporting framework of cells, contains the oocyte, lying to one side of the cavity, and itself surrounded by granulosa cells. Both these groups of cells are important sources of ovarian hormones, the oestrogens and progesterone.

Oestrogens These are hormones which govern the proliferative phase of the menstrual cycle, when the uterus thickens, the endometrium becoming more vascular and secretory. Changes also occur in the breasts and vagina, both becoming secretory. This lasts about 10 days.

Progesterone Progesterone further stimulates the endometrium, increasing its glandular activity. Breast glands also respond, causing premenstrual fullness and tingling. This secretory phase lasts 14 days and ends when the endometrium is shed, being redundant if fertilization has not occurred.

Ovulation

In response to a surge of activity by the luteinizing hormone, the follicular phase concludes with the rupture of the ripened graafian follicle onto the surface of the ovary (Fig. 2.9). The tension of the fluid within the follicle causes it to burst, and the oocyte is discharged with its surrounding cells into the peritoneum

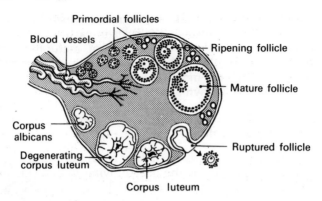

Fig. 2.9 **The sequence of changes occurring in the ovum during each menstrual cycle.**

to be conveyed onward by the fimbriae of the oviduct. This is known as ovulation and occurs at about the 14th day of the cycle (see Fig. 2.3). The growth of remaining follicles involved in the race to maturity is suppressed and they atrophy.

Luteal phase

Following ovulation, the luteal phase is concerned with the development and waning of a corpus luteum derived from the ruptured follicle. The remaining 'shell' of the follicle contains some granulosa and theca cells, which, under the influence of luteinizing hormone secrete progesterone every day for two weeks, then decreases in size unless the ovum is fertilized. The progesterone enriches the lining of the uterus. The corpus luteum, so named because it becomes swollen and yellow with fat (lutein—yellow pigment), retains some follicular fluid and fibrin. Its purpose is to 'tide over' the developing embryo by maintaining levels of progesterone until such time as the trophoblast, forerunner of the placenta, begins to provide its own. Naturally if no fertilization takes place, it is not needed, so begins to show signs of degeneration just before the onset of the next menstrual period. The reduction in output of progesterone brings on the menstrual flow— the haemorrhagic destruction of the superficial layers of the endometrium. The corpus luteum fibroses to become a shrunken white body, the corpus albicans.

If fertilization occurs, menstruation is inhibited by the maintenance of progesterone levels by the corpus luteum, which continues to develop, and may not degenerate until during the fifth month of pregnancy.

The luteal phase of the cycle is fairly constant, being 14 days in most women. There may be variations in the length of the pre-ovulatory or follicular stage in women, from seven to as much as 28 days. The menstrual flow, or menses, lasts from three to seven days, then a fresh cycle begins.

FERTILIZATION

Fertilization normally occurs in the fallopian tube. Vast numbers of sperm are contained in one ejaculate (about 3.5 ml of semen), but only one sperm penetrates the ovum. The ovum is covered with a protective layer, the zona pellucida, and as soon as one sperm has penetrated this layer, it undergoes changes which render the ovum impervious. If two sperm should succeed in penetrating the ovum, an abnormal conceptus results.

The sperm and the ovum each carry the full complement of each partner's genes, so that the conceptus or zygote formed at fertilization would have a double load unless half were shed. This process occurs at this stage, giving each individual his unique mix of parental genes. The zygote then begins the process of cell

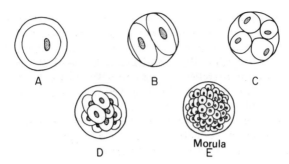

Fig. 2.10   A fertilized ovum undergoing cell division.

division, and then gradually starts to migrate towards the uterus. This takes about four to five days, by which time the zygote consists of about 30–50 cells and is called the morula (Fig. 2.10).

Implantation

The next important stage in the progress of the new pregnancy is implantation. The morula migrates to the uterine cavity and begins to embed itself in the proliferating endometrium, which has been becoming thicker and more richly supplied with blood vessels, in the hopes of welcoming a zygote. By the time implantation occurs, the morula has undergone changes in its cell arrangement, with some differentiation of cells, and is called a blastocyst. It is at this stage of development that further subdivision may occur, leading to the development of monozygotic twins. (Dizygotic twins result from the release and fertilization of two ova.) By about the seventh day after fertilization, the blastocyst has embedded in the endometrium. The various cells which have grouped themselves together will eventually develop into the placenta and membranes, and the fetus itself, with further cell differentiation and organization to form the different structures and systems. The group of cells forming the placenta includes the chorionic villi, which can be taken for microscopic examination, in order to detect certain abnormalities. The embryonic blood vessels begin to form by about day 14.

Failure of the zygote to implant is the cause of very early abortion, which may be unrecognized; it will appear as a late, rather heavy period.

Further development of the embryo

Detailed descriptions will not be given here, but it is important to remember that the embryonic systems are being formed in the earliest weeks of pregnancy, and that external factors—pollutants, bacteria and viruses, maternal drugs including alcohol and nicotine—can have an adverse effect on embryonic development during the first trimester (third) of pregnancy.

It is interesting to note one or two points:

At four weeks the embryo measures 1 cm in length, and consists of a head, tail fold and limb buds (Fig. 2.11).
At eight weeks the length is 5 cm.
At 12 weeks the length is 7.5 cm, and the fingernails are forming.
At 16 weeks the external genitalia can be identified, though of course sex was determined at conception. He or she is now 18 cm long.

As early as this all the vital systems are present and functioning, though of course they continue to develop and mature until 40 weeks, when the fetus is completely ready to function independently of the mother's body.

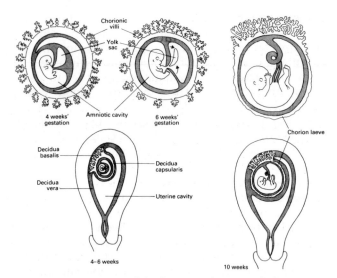

Fig. 2.11   Development of the fetus, membranes and placenta.

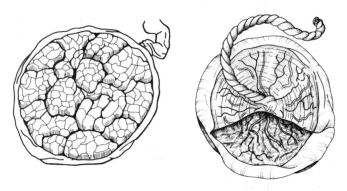

Fig. 2.12   The placenta. A, The maternal surface, B, The fetal surface.

The placenta (Fig. 2.12)

The placenta is an extremely important organ. It brings fetal blood to the uterine vessels, so that diffusion may occur from fetal to maternal blood and vice versa. Fetal and maternal blood do not actually mix, though in certain circumstances there may be spill-over of fetal cells. Substances diffused across the placental barrier by the 'concentration gradient' include oxygen, carbon dioxide, food products and waste matter. (When there is a concentration gradient across a permeable membrane, equilibrium is obtained on the two sides by the passage of a substance from the more concentrated to the less concentrated side.) By the same process, drugs are passed from mother to fetus. The factor determining whether or not substances can cross the 'placental barrier' is their molecular size. When the concentration gradient principle is in operation, as the mother's levels of, for example, a drug fall, so the fetus will diffuse the substance back for his mother's system to excrete, if his is unable to deal with it.

The link between fetus and placenta is the umbilical cord. This contains two umbilical arteries and one umbilical vein.

THE PHYSIOLOGY OF PREGNANCY

Maternal physiology and metabolism has to undergo considerable changes in order to support a growing fetus without compromising the mother's well-being. This is normally done very efficiently, as demonstrated by the majority of women, who 'bloom' in pregnancy, though most feel tired and often nauseated, in the first weeks.

The cardiovascular system

The blood volume must increase as pregnancy progresses, in order to service uterine and placental perfusion. The red cell content also increases, but not to the same extent, so there is a degree of haemodilution. The cardiac output obviously has to increase, but this is offset by a fall in peripheral resistance caused by progesterone effects (relaxing the plain muscle in the blood vessel walls). In fact a woman is often quite hypotensive in early pregnancy, explaining why some women are prone to fainting.

The gastrointestinal tract

Progesterone-induced changes affect the gastrointestinal tract in several ways. Gastric emptying is delayed, and with relaxed sphincters, nausea is a common complaint in early pregnancy, and heartburn in later pregnancy. Intestinal emptying is also slower, allowing the products of digestion to be absorbed to a greater degree. The relaxation of gut muscle causes constipation. The woman's metabolic needs will be greater, though 'eating for two' is definitely discouraged!

The renal system

Renal blood flow is increased, in order to transport the added waste products from the fetus. Progesterone affects the ureters, so that they become dilated and tortuous. Stasis of urine may lead to higher urinary tract infections—pyelitis and pyelonephritis. Cystitis is also commoner in pregnancy, and may cause ascending infection.

The glomerular filtration rate may increase by as much as 50% and this sometimes results in escape of glucose into the urine despite a blood sugar level within the normal range. Glycosuria in pregnancy may therefore not indicate abnormality, though it is always investigated.

The respiratory system

Tidal volume is increased in pregnancy, to cope with increased demand for gaseous exchange.

The breasts

Breast symptoms are some of the earliest in pregnancy, and it is during the first pregnancy that the final maturation of the breasts takes place.

Each breast, or mammary gland, consists of glands and ducts which are concerned with the manufacture and transport of milk. These are contained in separate lobes, rather like the segments of an orange. The glands and ducts are surrounded by fatty and connective tissue, and the whole structure is richly supplied with blood (Fig. 2.13).

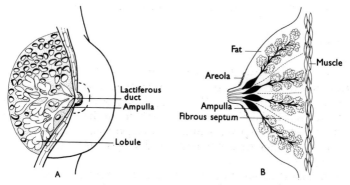

Fig. 2.13   The breast. A, The lobes seen from the front. B, Sagittal section.

The breasts both grow and develop in early pregnancy. The first symptom is often tingling or tenderness, and the first sign is enlargement. The nipples and areolae become enlarged, and usually darker. In darker skinned women with more pigmentation, the area around the areola may also darken; this is called the secondary areola. Around the nipple are small sebaceous glands which develop in the early weeks; these are called Montgomery's tubercles, and help protect the delicate skin of the nipple. The nipples should protract; that is, when compressed gently with a slight backward pressure, using the thumb and forefinger, the nipple should protrude, rather than retracting. Protraction usually improves to some extent as pregnancy progresses, and still further as the baby suckles, but treatment in the antenatal period may be helpful if nipples are flat or inverted. (See Chapter 17—'Infant Feeding'.)

The milk-producing cells, or acini, extract the necessary nutrients and constituents from the blood supply to the breast tissue. The cells group together to form glands. These drain into small ducts which converge to form a main duct, the lactiferous duct. The lactiferous duct widens out into a small reservoir, the ampulla, just behind the nipple. There is then a further small duct leading to the surface of the nipple.

PELVIC MEASUREMENTS

The mechanism of normal labour follows a clearly defined pattern, allowing the baby to follow the optimum route through the birth canal. In order to appreciate this, it is necessary to study the pelvic measurements and the diameters of the fetal skull, and relate the two.

The bony pelvis is described as consisting of the true

and the false pelvis. It is the 'true' pelvis which is of importance in obstetrics. The true pelvis consists of the brim, the cavity and the outlet, and in considering the dimensions of these, it is necessary to define the anteroposterior, transverse and oblique diameters. Each of these parts must be large enough to allow the fetus to pass through, but pelves vary in their proportions, and are classified accordingly (Fig. 2.14).

The typical female pelvis, which has each part well proportioned for childbirth, is called a 'gynaecoid' pelvis (see Table 2.1).

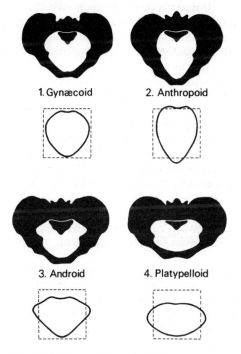

1. Gynæcoid   2. Anthropoid

3. Android   4. Platypelloid

Fig. 2.14 Inherited shapes of the pelvic brim.

Table 2.1   The measurements of a gynaecoid pelvis

	Antero posterior	Oblique	Transverse
Brim	11 cm	12 cm	13 cm
Cavity	12 cm	12 cm	12 cm
Outlet	13 cm	12 cm	11 cm

The 'anthropoid' pelvis has an oval brim, so that the anteroposterior diameter is reduced, and a long narrow sacrum. The anthropoid pelvis is often larger, so that vaginal delivery occurs without undue difficulty.

The typical male type of pelvis is called an 'android' pelvis. It has a triangular brim, a straight sacrum, and a smaller outlet. The woman with an android pelvis will have difficulty delivering anything other than a small baby spontaneously.

The 'platypelloid' or flat pelvis is flattened anteroposteriorly.

The pelvic brim is readily defined on a model pelvis (Fig. 2.15). Its landmarks are:

the sacral promontory
the alae (wings) of the sacrum
the sacro-iliac joint
the ilio-pectineal line
the ilio-pectineal eminence
the upper, inner border of the superior pubic rami
the upper, inner border of the pubic symphysis

If an imaginary line links all these points on both sides of the pelvis, the pelvic brim can be understood.

The pelvic cavity is defined by the sacrum posteriorly and the pubic symphysis anteriorly. If drawn in sagittal section, it is seen to be long posteriorly, and short anteriorly. This means that the birth canal follows a curve. The soft tissues of the birth canal also follow this

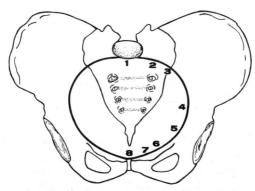

Fig. 2.15 The pelvic brim. 1, promontory of the sacrum; 2, ala of the sacrum; 3, sacro-iliac joint; 4, ilio-pectineal line; 5, ilio-pectineal eminence; 6, superior pubic ramus; 7, body of pubic bone; 8, symphysis pubis.

curve, since the uterus is at right angles to the vagina. This is called the curve of Carus.

The pelvic outlet is defined by the lower sacrum and the pubic arch.

As the fetus passes through the pelvis, its passage is aided by the fact that the fetal head moulds, that is, the skull bones override each other slightly. The pelvis also enlarges slightly, as one of the effects of progesterone is to soften the ligaments. If the woman delivers in one of the 'alternative' positions (see Chapter 11—'Normal Labour'), the coccyx is more mobile, so that the outlet enlarges slightly more.

THE FETAL SKULL

Certain points on the fetal skull form important landmarks for the midwife and obstetrician, and give rise to the names of the various diameters.

The fetal skull consists of seven bones; embryo-logically these develop from membrane, and ossify from the centre during intrauterine life. The ossification process has developed sufficiently at term to protect the head, but not to the extent that the skull bones cannot override each other slightly during labour—the process of moulding.

Some definitions

Suture—the line felt between two bones in the skull.
Fontanelle—the gap felt where more than two skull bones meet. A fontanelle is covered with membrane.
Mentum—the chin.
Bregma—the anterior fontanelle.
Vertex—the name given to the area between the anterior and posterior fontanelles, which presents in a normal delivery.

The bones of the fetal skull (Figs. 2.16 and 2.17)

The facial bones are not considered in this context, as they do not have any obstetric significance.
The bones of the vault are:

two frontal bones
two parietal bones
two temporal bones
one occipital bone

The sutures

The *lambdoidal suture* runs between the parietal bones and the occipital bone.
The *sagittal suture* runs between the two parietal bones.

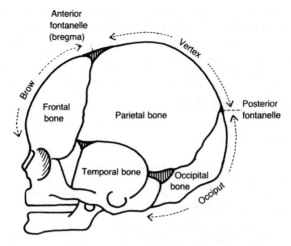

Fig. 2.16   The bones, fontanelles and regions of the fetal skull.

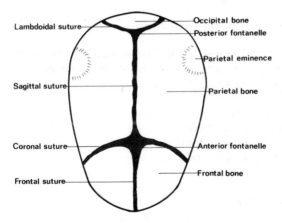

Fig. 2.17   The fetal skull, showing the bones, fontanelles and sutures.

The *coronal suture* runs between the parietal and frontal bones.

The fontanelles

The *anterior fontanelle* or bregma is situated where the sagittal and coronal sutures cross; it lies at the junction of four bones, the frontal and parietal bones. It closes at about 18 months of age.

The *posterior fontanelle* lies at the junction of three bones, the occipital and two parietal bones.

The diameters of the fetal skull (Fig. 2.18)

The significant diameter of the fetal skull is that one which is at right angles to the birth canal during delivery. In a normal delivery the smallest diameter, the suboccipitobregmatic, is passing through the birth canal, because the head is flexed.

When a baby presents by the brow, the largest diameter would have to pass through the birth canal, and so a brow presentation cannot be delivered vaginally. (The largest diameter is the mentovertical.)

The diameters are:

suboccipitobregmatic: 9.5 cm
suboccipitofrontal: 10 cm
occipitofrontal: 11.5 cm
mentovertical: 13.5 cm
submentovertical: 11 cm
submentobregmatic: 9.5 cm

There are also two lateral diameters:

biparietal: 9.5 cm—measured between the widest points on the two parietal bones
bitemporal: 8 cm

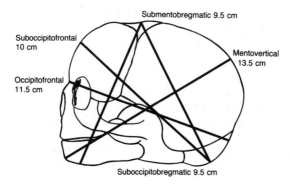

Fig 2.18   The diameters of the fetal skull.

Moulding

As already described, this is the process whereby the skull bones override each other slightly in order to facilitate the fetus's passage through the birth canal.

It should not be excessive, nor occur rapidly, since there is then a danger of damage to the underlying structures—the cerebral membranes, which have blood vessels running through them; these will rupture if the membranes are torn.

Optimum moulding occurs during normal labour, with a well-flexed head.

FURTHER READING

BURNETT, C. W. F. (1969) *The Anatomy and Physiology of Obstetrics*, 5th edn. London: Faber & Faber.

FLLIS, H. (1979) *Clinical Anatomy*, 4th edn. Oxford: Blackwell Scientific Publications.

LLEWELLYN-JONES, D. (1982) *Fundamentals of Obstetrics and Gynaecology*, Vol. 1 3rd edn. London: Faber & Faber.

Moore, K. L. (1983) *Before We Are Born* (Basic Embryology and Birth Defects). W. B. Saunders.

Ross, J. S. & Wilson, K. J. W. (1982) *Foundations of Anatomy and Physiology*, 5th edn. Edinburgh: Churchill Livingstone.

3

WOMEN AND SEXUALITY

Sexuality may be defined as the becoming and being of a woman or a man. It involves a self-concept or self-worth, and a person's view of the body in relation to other people. It means a certain acceptance of feminine and masculine gender roles. Sexuality then, is more than biology; it is a quality of being human, and how to express this.

ASPECTS OF SEXUALITY

In terms of definitions, the word 'sex' is usually applied to the biological aspects of sexuality, and 'gender' is applied to the social aspects. An individual's physical attributes are based on the genotype—XX or XY—but expression of her or his sexuality does not necessarily depend on it.

Gender, relating to the culture in which a person is brought up, has much to do with learned behaviour.

Gender stereotypes are personality characteristics which are believed to be appropriate for women and men. Such stereotyping is said to be built up from infancy, and there has been considerable interest shown in how parents treat their female and male offspring. It is generally thought that the majority of parents treat boys and girls differently, although this may be unconscious. For example, in British society boys are not encouraged to cry and girls tend to be encouraged in female pursuits such as playing with dolls and imitating housework. However, schools are more conscious nowadays of such stereotypes and try to eliminate them where possible.

Gender roles are given to women and men by particular cultures who define what is appropriate. This means that in European societies men do the 'heavy' work, women the housework. In many developing countries it is the exclusive task of women to fetch water.

Gender identity relates to how a person defines herself or himself as a sexual being, i.e. heterosexual, homosexual, bisexual etc. To have—and be known to have— a gender identity is vital for most people. This is shown by the importance which 'coming out' to her or his family and friends has for a homosexual.

Gender preference is the attraction a person has to other people and with whom she or he prefers to have sexual relations.

Volumes have been written on these aspects of sexuality down the centuries. If history could be written in terms of sexuality, it would be obvious that nothing drives humanity as much as love (and money) and how to have them. Indeed, some writers have placed both the rise of sexual repression and homosexual liberation into the context of the development of capitalism, (e.g. Foucault in the seventeenth century, Snitow, Stansell & Thompson in the 1960s).

EXPRESSION OF SEXUALITY

From the times of cave dwellers to the present, artists have captured sexuality in its many forms. Sexuality is expressed all day and every day by the way people dress, talk, walk, relate to friends and strangers.

The five senses are essential to the expression of

sexuality, both in genital contact and in everyday relationships. Yet humans seem to be the only mammals who can be sexually aroused by the mind alone. Indeed, the saying 'the mind is the major sex organ of the (human) body' is not too far fetched.

The way in which a person expresses her or his sexuality varies greatly and depends on all the above factors. Health or illness may additionally enhance or jeopardize this expression.

Until fairly recently the only legitimate form of sexual expression was heterosexual. Other forms were labelled as deviant and were banished. Homosexuality between consenting men aged 21 years and over was legalized in 1967, and since then other types of sexuality have become more acceptable too. It is now estimated that 1 in 10 men are preferentially homosexual (although not necessarily sexually active) and that 1 in 4 men have had a homosexual experience at some stage in their lives.

Lesbianism has never been illegal in the United Kingdom due to Queen Victoria's refusal to believe in the existence of homosexuality between women, and yet an estimated 10% of women are lesbian.

Bisexuality—enjoying sexual relations with women and men—is less often mentioned in literature; such a person can be less easily 'labelled'.

Transsexuals are persons of either male or female genotype who feel and experience themselves as of the opposite type. Through sex change operations and hormone therapy they can live in that gender. Legally, however, a person cannot become a member of the opposite sex, and is not able to marry.

Transvestites are almost always men who are sexually aroused by wearing women's clothes.

Celibates are women and men who have either chosen or been forced (by circumstances) to remain sexually inactive.

Within these groupings, sexual activity can vary

greatly. It can be by 'a variety of partners, or alone; using a variety of techniques in a variety of circumstances'.

The present relaxation of censure on sexual activity and expression is conditioned by centuries of repression. This does not mean that overtones of sin, guilt, fear of being found out and any number of accusations from within a person and from society have disappeared too. People who express themselves sexually in 'unusual' ways are as sensitive to disapproval as anyone who dares to differ in any way.

Women are still largely considered to be 'the weaker sex' by men; the ones who incite men; the ones who are always underneath. As many women begin to throw off the shackles of all kinds of stereotypes, they liberate themselves also from *sexual* stereotypes. Some women, however, still prefer to retain their 'traditional' roles.

THE PHYSIOLOGY OF THE SEXUAL RESPONSE

It is important to appreciate the factors affecting female sexual response, its nature, and how it differs from the male response (though the latter will not be discussed in detail in this text).

The physiology of sexual response is described under four headings.

1. Excitement phase   This occurs as a result of various stimuli including mental images and fantasies. The most important stimulus for the woman is touch whereas a man is more readily aroused by what he sees. The most sensitive areas for the woman are the clitoris, labia and vagina, but almost the whole of her body responds positively to caressing. The excitement phase tends to be longer for women than for men. As sexual arousal takes place the vagina starts to become moist, partly as a result of transudate from the engorging blood vessels, and partly from the Bartholin's glands at the introitus. The labia and clitoris become engorged and swollen and the nipples become erect.

2. Plateau phase   As foreplay continues sexual excitement mounts. The vagina is well lubricated and the introitus is swollen and open.

3. Orgasmic phase   An intensely pleasurable sensation engulfs the whole body. The vagina and vulva feel particularly sensitive, the uterus contracts rhythmically as do the vaginal muscles and many of the skeletal muscles.

4. Resolution phase   The sexual excitement dies down gradually, leaving the woman pleasantly relaxed and sleepy. At this point, with continued stimulation a woman may experience further orgasms, unlike a man.

How, when and where the sexual act is effected will vary greatly. Most women associate sex with love and a need for relationship and security. But how and with whom they achieve this is less and less bound by convention.

SEXUALITY AND WOMEN IN THE NURSING CONTEXT

Kuczynski noted that in 1973 the World Health Organization (WHO) found 'that little relevant teaching of human sexuality was offered in most nursing and medical schools throughout the world'. What teaching was provided tended to be on 'reproductive physiology, orientation to family relationships and some preparation to interviewing'. However, this did not include the student's own understanding of her or his sexuality, the psychological and social aspects of procreation, and the implications of a rapidly increasing population. Small wonder that nurses tend to 'avoid counselling situations or counsel with decreased sensitivity, objectivity and empathy'. Fear and prejudice lie at the root of many of these difficulties, but also the nursing culture, tradition, and perhaps a reluctance to change. Furthermore, despite the fact that an estimated 1 in 10 women are lesbian, a North American survey conducted in 1985 revealed that 'low grade homophobia' (fear of homosexuality) was exhibited by nurses and doctors working in a large teaching hospital. Such homophobia is also present in the UK health service and it is vital that nurses begin to familiarize themselves with sexuality in its fullest sense in order to deliver effective, holistic care from a non-judgemental and sensitive standpoint.

With greater emphasis on holistic care and primary nursing, and the implications of Project 2000 (the new approach to pre-registration nurse education in the United Kingdom), the priorities of dealing with patients must be a regard and respect for the whole person, her or his understanding of the illness or disease and participation in the healing process.

Admission procedures and treatments given in areas of obstetrics and gynaecology need to reflect the sensitive nature of the problems involved. In particular, the standard forms and questions used in many instances should be questioned and examined for their relevance. Questions such as the nature of a person's marital status, next-of-kin, or use of contraceptives can be value-laden, sexist, and insensitive. How and where patients are interviewed can make the difference between cooperation with or suspicion of care and treatment. Hospital policies, particularly with regard to who is entitled to have information about the patient, may also need to be questioned. They may be not only irrelevant but particularly hurtful—e.g. in the case of a lesbian couple—in an already sensitive position. Finally, how patients are examined is of the greatest importance. To the nurse it may not be more than a procedure, but the patient will see it from a different standpoint. Exposing the most intimate part of herself to one, or possibly several, strangers who then may confirm an illness to her, is demanding for anyone. If a patient's fears and embarrassment can be gently dealt with and respected, both parties will feel more satisfied.

BODY IMAGE

'Our body provides the basis for understanding our personal world' says Savage. Making sense of one's personal world seems to be most people's major task in life. When this is brought more sharply into focus, through illness, bereavement—or indeed through having a baby—the body becomes more important. The image a person has of her body becomes more related to self-worth and self-concept in general.

A person's body image can be drastically altered by disease and illness, or through accidents, surgery, or age. But how that person's body image was before any interference will colour how she responds during and after any trauma.

Many people go through life with a low self-concept. Any visible mark or congenital abnormality such as being small, or tall, having large breasts, a high voice, or any deformity 'can make people insecure in their body image and aware that others may think of them as "abnormal", and this may make them feel unwanted as friends and sexual partners'.

Mutilating surgery, such as mastectomy and ileostomy or colostomy, are well recognized in causing difficulties for patients. Other less 'obvious' operations

may cause deep scars emotionally even if not physically. Episiotomy, hysterectomy, caesarean section may
all alter a person's self-image considerably. Stretch-
marks, 'middle-age spread', abortion, herpes, having,
or being afraid of having, HIV, loss of hair from chemotherapy and many other aspects can be the cause
of tension, loss of self-worth, general ill health and
worry. Patients may keep these anxieties to themselves,
through shame, disgust at themselves, or helplessness.

A nurse who is sensitive to these issues and possible
problems may not only help the patient to a recovery,
but to wholeness. Being attentive, listening rather than
talking, touching and demonstrating affection convey
an empathy which may be just as necessary as any
medication.

SEXUAL PROBLEMS

Some of the more common sexual problems need also
to be mentioned.

'*Frigidity*' is the term used for a woman who is unable
to respond sexually and may hate being touched or
fondled. She may never have experienced orgasm,
or the condition may be secondary to a traumatic
experience.

Loss of libido (sexual desire) is common at certain
points in a woman's life, such as in the months following childbirth. It can also be caused by medication,
such as antihistamines, narcotics and cytotoxics.

Ill health, anorexia, repeated cystitis and hormone
imbalance may all be physical causes of lack of libido.
Emotional causes are perhaps just as common, such as
fear of pregnancy, a poor body image and disharmony
in the relationship with the sexual partner.

Dyspareunia, or painful intercourse, may be deep
or superficial. This is a common complaint in the

gynaecology clinic, although a woman may find it difficult to admit to it initially, and may be embarrassed to discuss it. The physical causes may be superficial or deep.

Superficial: painful episiotomy scar, Bartholinitis, infections such as herpes, vaginitis, lack of vaginal lubrication, vaginal atrophy (usually postmenopausal).

Deep: cervicitis, endometriosis, pelvic inflammatory disease and possibly urinary problems such as cystitis.

The emotional causes for this problem are similar to those mentioned above under loss of libido.

Vaginismus is a condition in which the vagina goes into spasm on any attempt to penetrate the introitus, whether during digital or penile penetration or pelvic examination. The woman will probably be unable to use tampons. The basis of this problem is often fear, which may be well-founded or irrational.

These commonly mentioned sexual problems may increase with age, particularly during and after the menopause when changes in the sex organs take place. With sensitivity—and excluding physical problems or disease—a person may be encouraged to view sexuality in less stereotyped ways, and other forms and positions of sexual expression may be encouraged. Psychosexual counselling or sex therapy may be one way to help a person. This may involve a long-term commitment and may involve wide-ranging investigation into the client's background, upbringing, past relationships, and any previous problems. It may require a variety of techniques in order to help an individual. It is usually done with the client's partner since one person's difficulties will affect the whole relationship.

CONCLUSION

Sexuality is at the basis of obstetric and gynaecological nursing care. For that care to be holistic, sexuality needs to be seen as far more than just a biological function. For a nurse to understand and help her or his patient, she or he needs to be 'in touch' with the whole of the patient—which may occasionally present a challenge, and will always lead to health and satisfaction.

FURTHER READING

FOUCAULT, M. (1978) *The History of Sexuality*. Harmondsworth; Penguin.

GLOVER, J. (1985) *Human Sexuality in Nursing Care*. London: Croom Helm.

JONES, R. (1988) With respect to lesbians. *Nursing Times*, **84** (20), 48–49.

KINSEY, A. (1953) *Sexual Behaviour in the Human Female*. Philadelphia, W. B. Saunders.

KUCZYNSKI, J. (1986) Liberal studies. *Nursing Times*, **32** (28), 60–61.

OAKLEY, A. (1972) *Sex, Gender and Society*. London: Temple Smith.

SAVAGE, J. (1987) *Nurses, Gender and Sexuality*. London: Heinemann.

SNITOW, A., STANSELL, C. & THOMPSON, S. (1984) *Desire—the Politics of Sexuality*. London. Virago.

TIEFER, L. (1979) *Human Sexuality*. London: Harper & Row.

WEBB, C. (1985) *Sexuality, Nursing and Health*. Chichester, John Wiley.

WEBB, C. (1987) Sexual healing. *Nursing Times*, **83** (32), 29–30.

Obstetrics

4

PREPARATION FOR PARENTHOOD

ROLE DEFINITIONS AND EXPECTATIONS

Preparation for parenthood begins early in life, as expectations, and social and cultural norms and values are consciously and subconsciously absorbed. Psychologists and sociologists have devoted considerable time and effort to studying gender roles, and whether or not parents treat girl and boy babies differently, and therefore make them different.

Emerging from all their findings is the indisputable fact that human beings are complex creatures, and that the whole subject of sex and gender roles, and what factors influence our arriving at our own concept of these, is still wide open for debate.

Probably the next stage in preparation for parenthood is an assimilation of one's own parents' attitudes and parental behaviour, which tends then to be repeated in the next generation. Certainly the 'cycle of deprivation' theory, and the fact that child abuse tends to repeat itself in a family would seem to bear out this suggestion.

With the widening of the social circle, as a child attends playgroup and then school, comes a wider appreciation of values.

SEX EDUCATION

This is a much debated topic. There would seem to be a joint responsibility, shared by the family and the school. However, there is still much coyness and embarrassment in evidence, despite much freer and open attitudes, as well as much ignorance and many old wives' tales. There is an unfortunate tendency to concentrate on the mechanical aspects of sex and contraception, and to fail to attempt to communicate the importance of caring, responsible relationships, and the emotional aspect of sexuality.

The importance of being caring and responsible in a sexual relationship should then lead on naturally to planning to become parents in a thoughtful and responsible fashion. However, this is a starry-eyed ideal at present, and despite the fact that contraception is so easily available, there are many reluctant parents.

PRECONCEPTUAL CARE

A decade or two ago, antenatal care was seen as the ideal means of ensuring a healthy mother and baby. To a certain extent this is true, but the provision of antenatal care has not solved every problem, or reduced the perinatal mortality rate as much as had been hoped.

In fact, the antenatal period is too late for some preventive measures, and so in some centres, preconceptual care is offered. Responsibly planned parenthood is not just a question of seeking contraceptive advice, but of ensuring that both parents are fit and healthy. Smoking has been shown to have an adverse effect on placental function, and if a woman can reduce or give up smoking before becoming pregnant, so much the better. Alcohol consumption is an even more important issue, since large amounts of alcohol have been shown to have an adverse effect on organogenesis—before many women are aware they are pregnant, and certainly before they have sought antenatal care. A healthy diet is an important consideration too, and also the avoidance of pollutants and occupational hazards where relevant. Testing women for immunity to rubella before they plan to start a family enables them to accept immunization if necessary. Rubella in early pregnancy may lead to a child being born with a variety of impairments, such as blindness, deafness and mental handicap.

Advice is simply given in a family planning clinic, if the nurse knows her clients well, by the health visitor, and in 'well woman' clinics. It could well be taken up by the media, and such matters are frequently aired in women's magazines.

Recognizing that even the antenatal booking appointment is too late for some aspects of health education in preparation for parenthood, some feel that the antenatal services should expand to provide a 'walk in' pregnancy testing service. Women with positive results could then be booked immediately for antenatal care.

Another aspect of preconceptual care, however, has to do with women with an underlying medical problem, such as diabetes, or cardiac or renal problems. In many centres, obstetricians and physicians work closely together, and run joint clinics. This enables the doctors to manage both aspects of the woman's care, without giving conflicting advice, and without asking her to attend too many extra out-patient clinics.

Some drug regimens may need to be modified if pregnancy is planned. It has been shown that well-controlled diabetes before conception leads to a better outcome for both mother and baby. The physically handicapped woman may need expert advice and counselling before she and her partner decide to embark on a pregnancy. Similarly, the couple with a family history of hereditary disease or abnormality may need genetic counselling.

FURTHER READING

BOURNE, G. (1975) *Pregnancy*. London: Pan Books.

CHAMBERLAIN, G. (1990) *Preparing for Pregnancy*. London: Fontana Collins.

CHAMBERLAIN, G. & LUMLEY, J. (1986) *Pre-Pregnancy Care*. Chichester: John Wiley.

DALLY, A. (1982) *Inventing Motherhood*. London: Burnett Books.

5

FERTILITY CONTROL

Women in the 1990s have more control over their
fertility than ever before. Recent advances in *in vitro*
fertilization (IVF) mean that the previously infertile
woman with no chance of becoming pregnant now has
some hope.

Fertility control therefore does not only imply the
prevention of conception, but also embraces the whole
field of subfertility and infertility.

INFERTILITY

As many as 10% of couples fail to achieve a pregnancy
without some kind of medical help, and the problem
may lie with either partner.

A woman may suffer from primary infertility, in
which case she has never been fertile.

She may have been pregnant in the past, but subsequently been unable to conceive again; this is called
secondary infertility. The problem may be due to:

Poor or absent ovarian function because of some
abnormality of either the ovaries themselves, or the
pituitary gland.
A mechanical factor, such as blocked fallopian tubes.
A common cause of this is pelvic inflammatory
disease.
'Hostile' mucus in the vagina or cervix which may
impede the progress of sperm.

Fibroids—these may tend to prevent implantation of the zygote.

Similarly the man may have a problem with the production of sperm, or with some obstruction of the seminal ducts.

There may be some form of sexual dysfunction in either partner, preventing full, effective intercourse.

A couple who are being investigated for infertility are subjected to investigations of a very personal nature. They will have been questioned closely about their sexual activity. Only a couple who very much want a baby are likely to stay the course! They suffer profound disappointment every month. Happily, many couples find that they only need to be referred for help, and the woman becames pregnant shortly afterwards.

Investigations

For the woman:

Measurement of hormone levels—progesterone, gonadotrophin, prolactin.

Temperature chart—the morning temperature rises around the time of ovulation.

Examination of cervical mucus—this shows typical changes around ovulation.

Dilatation and curettage to examine the endometrium.

Laparoscopy—to examine the fallopian tubes and the ovaries.

Hysterosalpingogram to test for tubal patency.

For the man:

Semen analysis—a sperm count shows both the number and the nature of the sperm; if fertilization is to be a realistic hope the sperm must be normal, mature and of sufficient number.

Measurement of hormone levels—gonadotrophin.

For both:

Postcoital test—the pool of semen lying around the cervix is aspirated and examined for numbers of healthy, motile sperm. This is done within an hour or two of intercourse.

Treatment

Treatment for the woman may involve tubal surgery or the use of 'fertility drugs'.

The so-called fertility drugs stimulate ovulation, and hormone levels must then be monitored carefully so as to avoid multiple pregnancies with more than two fetuses.

Artificial insemination—this may involve the use of the husband's semen or that of a donor—AIH or AID.

In vitro fertilization (IVF)—the so-called 'test tube baby'.

Gamete intrafallopian transfer (GIFT)

Hormone implants, to stimulate the pituitary gland in women with poor ovarian function, seem to be a possibility in the near future.

Ethics and dilemmas

Medical advances usually bring some kind of ethical dilemma. The Warnock Report was set up to investigate the whole area of fertility control, looking at matters such as the storage of embryos, their use for research, and surrogate motherhood, for example. At the time of writing the Embryo Research Bill is being debated in the UK Parliament.

CONTRACEPTION

The general practitioner may provide contraceptive services for his or her patients, or the woman may prefer to attend a Family Planning Clinic. Nurses working in these clinics are specially trained in family planning, and are in a good position to get to know their clients well, gain their trust, and to offer advice and health education. The woman who has just had a baby will also be offered family planning advice, and this will be followed up at her postnatal check, six weeks after the birth.

At the present time, contraception is available free of charge. Sheaths and spermicidal preparations may be purchased in chemists. They may be obtained free from the Family Planning Clinic, but not from the general practitioner. However, there are thoughts of making sheaths more available from the general practitioner, in an attempt to reduce the spread of AIDS.

Methods

No method of contraception is 100% reliable, and couples must be advised of this.

Barrier methods   These do not affect ovulation, but prevent sperm and ovum from meeting. These methods have become more popular in recent years because they do not involve any physiological changes, and the only complications are possible failure and allergy to the rubber or the spermicide. (Some condoms are impregnated with spermicide; those which are not

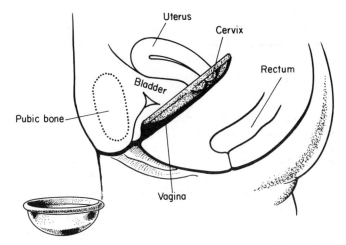

Fig. 5.1 The diaphragm cap in position.

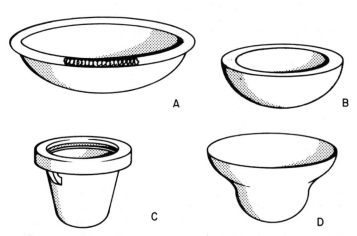

Fig. 5.2 Occlusive caps. A, Diaphragm. B, Vault cap. C, Cervical cap. D, Vimule cap.

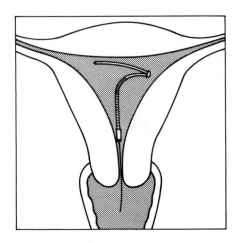

Fig. 5.3   IUCD in place.

should be used with a separate spermicidal preparation.) For the woman the barrier method involves the
use of a cap (Fig. 5.1), and for the man, the condom
or sheath.

There are various types of cap (Fig. 5.2):

'flat' and 'coil spring' diaphragms
'arcing' diaphragm
cervical cap
vault cap
vimule

The woman is taught how to use the cap, whichever
type she is given.

Spermicides These are available as cream, foam,
jelly or pessaries and couples are advised to use them
in conjunction with one of the barrier methods.

The intrauterine contraceptive device or IUCD (Fig. 5.3) This method is thought to inhibit implantation of the fertilized ovum, and some couples will object to its use on these grounds, as it can therefore be argued that it is an abortifacient. It may cause menorrhagia for some women, and there is a very slight risk of pelvic infection.

There are different types of IUCD:

inert (plastic)
copper
medicated

'The pill' These work by inhibiting ovulation, and contain a combination of oestrogen and progesterone. Women taking 'the pill' are monitored carefully. There is an element of risk in women with hypertension, varicose veins, who are obese, or who smoke. They are probably more likely to develop thromboembolic disorders, or suffer a myocardial infarction or a cerebrovascular accident. Most doctors prescribe 'the pill' for older women, aged 35 years or over, with some caution particularly if they have been taking it for many years. However, there is now a low dose combined pill containing less oestrogen, and this may be prescribed for older women who are 'low risk': those who do not smoke, have no adverse medical history and are not obese.

The 'progesterone only' pill is a little different, in that it acts on the cervical mucus, making it hostile to sperm, and making the uterine environment less receptive to the fertilized ovum. It provides less reliable contraception and must be taken at the same time each day. It is useful for some women who could be at risk taking the combined pill, and for women who are breast-feeding.

'Natural family planning' This involves using the 'safe period', when ovulation is unlikely, for intercourse. The Billings method involves teaching women to recognize changes in their vaginal mucus, and from this, to predict ovulation. The other means of recognizing ovulation is by recording the morning temperature, and the woman is taught to do this before she gets out of bed each morning. When charted, a typical rise is seen around ovulation. These methods have a positive application for the woman who wishes to conceive.

Depo Provera injection   It is possible to give an intramuscular injection of progesterone which will be effective for three to six months. Another preparation, Noristerat, is effective for about eight weeks. Women may suffer from amenorrhoea or irregular bleeding.

Postcoital contraception   This is commonly known as 'morning after' contraception, though the preferred term now is emergency contraception. This may be available to women who have unprotected intercourse, if they seek help soon afterwards. One method is to give two large doses of the contraceptive pill 12 hours apart, within 72 hours of unprotected intercourse; the woman may feel very nauseated. The other method is to fit an IUCD within five days. Neither method is recommended as anything other than an emergency measure.

Sterilization   This is available to both men and women. Couples should be advised that it is permanent; although it may be possible to reverse the surgery, the chances of success are not very great. Female sterilization involves ligating or clipping the fallopian tubes (Fig. 5.4); this is frequently performed via the laparoscope nowadays. Occasionally it may be performed abdominally in the immediate postnatal period, but this is not without risk, and is less reliable. Women usually describe mixed feelings after tubal ligation, even when they were certain that they did not want

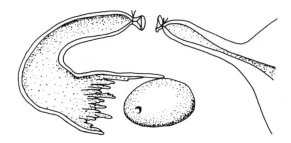

Fig. 5.4   Ligation of the fallopian tubes.

any more children. A degree of depression, and sometimes guilt, is quite common. The nurse needs to be
aware of this, and be prepared to support and reassure
the woman.

Male sterilization is performed by ligating the vas
deferens (Fig. 5.5), and may be performed under local
anaesthetic without the need for hospital admission.

Other methods   There are various other methods,
which are not reliable, and are not officially recommended. They include:

C-film (nonoxynol-9)
the sponge—a vaginal sponge containing spermicide
the 'honey' sponge

The future

With the potential complications of using the pill,
there is continual research aimed at finding the ideal
contraceptive. A slow-release progesterone implant,
vaginal rings and skin patches are possibilities under
investigation. There is a feeling among some women
that men should take greater responsibility for fertility
control, and researchers are interested in the possibility
of a 'male pill'.

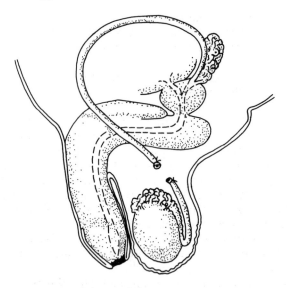

Fig. 5.5 Ligation of the vas deferens.

TERMINATION OF PREGNANCY

This topic is also discussed in Chapter 9.—'Problems in Early Pregnancy'.

It is not appropriate to regard termination of pregnancy as a means of fertility control, but there is always the feeling that it is available as an emergency measure if all else fails.

Since the introduction of the Abortion Act of 1967, it has been possible for women in the UK to have a pregnancy terminated without too much difficulty. The Act states that two doctors must examine the woman, and agree that the continuation of her pregnancy would place her at greater risk than if it were terminated, taking into account the following factors:

The life of the mother.
The physical or mental health of the mother.
The physical or mental health of any other child or children.
The substantial risk of serious physical or mental abnormality in the baby.

The two doctors must then sign a form to this effect. The Act also states that termination of pregnancy may only be carried out in approved institutions.

It is difficult for a woman who is very upset about being pregnant to appreciate the long-term implications of having her pregnancy terminated, however well she is counselled. However, counselling is very important, and she should have all the possible alternative options explained to her. The problem is that time is short; the earlier abortion is carried out, the better.

The nurse needs to appreciate that the woman is likely to feel guilty and depressed at some stage; this may not emerge fully until she is pregnant again. Many women will have mixed feelings about having an abortion. Many would prefer not to take this course of action, but are doing what they feel best. The nurse must support the woman in her decision, whatever her own personal feelings may be. Trained staff need to be aware of the need to offer support to their colleagues when necessary.

There is also the risk of damage to the cervix, so that it becomes incompetent in subsequent pregnancies.

Methods

Vacuum aspiration   This is the usual method used in the first trimester of pregnancy.

Prostaglandin   This may be administered by the intra- or extra-amniotic route. It can be a long, slow, painful experience, and very traumatic for a young teenager, for example.

Hysterotomy With the wide use of prostaglandin, this method is now rarely used. It carries the attendant risks of anaesthesia in pregnancy, and a scarred uterus is at risk of rupturing in a subsequent labour.

SEX AND THE UNDER-16s

This was a controversial topic in the mid 1980s, when Victoria Gillick protested strongly about doctors prescribing the contraceptive pill without parents' knowledge and consent. This had important implications for general practitioners and their young patients about confidentiality, and generated strong feelings on both sides of the debate. There were fears that the number of pregnancies in young teenagers would rise dramatically, but this did not happen. Although this controversy did die down it raised important issues and dilemmas for doctors and nurses involved in family planning.

Both the Royal College of General Practitioners and the Family Planning Association issued guidelines to medical and nursing staff involved in providing contraceptive services. The guidelines enabled staff to maintain young people's nights to confidentiality but encouraged the involvement of parents. Girls were to be counselled about the implications of becoming sexually active at a young age, but were to be prescribed the contraceptive pill if it was likely they were risking an unwanted pregnancy.

FURTHER READING

BAYLES. M. D. (1984) *Reproductive Ethics*. Prentice Hall Series in the Philosophy of Medicine.

BILLINGS, E. & WESTMORE, A. (1981) *The Billings Method*. Harmondsworth: Penguin Books.

COWPER, A. & YOUNG, C. (1981) *Family Planning*. London: Croom Helm.

GUILLEBAUD, J. (1983) *The Pill*. Oxford University Press.

LOUDEN, N. (1985) *Handbook of Family Planning*. Edinburgh: Churchill Livingstone.

PEPPERELL, R. J., HUDSON, B., & WOOD, C. (1980) *The Infertile Couple*. Edinburgh: Churchill Livingstone.

6

NORMAL PREGNANCY

SOME TERMS AND DEFINITIONS

The student nurse will find a whole new range of terms and abbreviations in use when she starts she obstetric experience. A more comprehensive list appears in the glossary on page 423, but a few may be helpful here.

Gravidity This refers to the number of pregnancies a woman has had, whatever their outcome. Thus a pregnancy, for example, which ends in spontaneous abortion at eight weeks, is included in gravidity.

Parity This refers to the number of viable children a woman has borne, whether or not they are still alive.

Viability This is a legal concept, in the early 1990s a controversial one. It refers to the ability of the infant to sustain life outside the uterus, and since the introduction of the term, a viable infant in the UK has been defined as one being born after 28 weeks' gestation. With improved neonatal intensive care, however, many babies born before the 28th week now survive, and grow into healthy children. Other countries define viability as occurring after 22 or 24 weeks' gestation, but this is still the subject of debate in the UK.

A primigravida, then, is a woman who is pregnant for the first time.

A primipara is a woman who has borne one child.

Similarly a multigravida is pregnant for the second or subsequent time. A multipara has borne two or more children. A grande multipara is usually defined as a woman who has borne four or more children.

An elderly primigravida is variously defined as a woman of anything from 25 years upwards, who is pregnant for the first time. This definition is based on the theory that the optimum childbearing years are from 18 to 24, but many women in Britain are now becoming pregnant later in life, and the term should be used with discretion!

In obstetric jargon a woman may be described as 'gravida 2 para 1' (abbreviated to 'Gr2 P1') if she is pregnant for the second time, having had one child. If her first pregnancy had ended in spontaneous abortion, she would be described as 'Gr2 P0'. If her first pregnancy had been a twin pregnancy, she would be described as 'Gr2 P2'.

LMP stands for 'last menstrual period', and the expected date of delivery (EDD) is calculated from the first day of the last normal period. The EDD may also be referred to as the EDC—expected date of confinement.

HOW A WOMAN KNOWS

Amenorrhoea The most obvious sign of pregnancy is amenorrhoea, and for women with a consistently regular cycle, this may be a very early indication.

Breast changes Associated with this are the breast changes already described in Chapter 2; initially tenderness and tingling, followed by enlargement.

Frequency of micturition The woman may complain of frequency of micturition as the enlarging uterus presses on the bladder.

Other symptoms include tiredness, and nausea or vomiting, usually, though not always, on waking in the mornings.

Some women 'feel' pregnant, instinctively knowing that they are. A 'phantom pregnancy', or pseudocyesis, may occur if a woman is excessively anxious either to become or not become pregnant. In this case, any or all of the signs and symptoms of pregnancy may be present, including an increase in abdominal girth, but all conclusive tests will of course remain negative. The mind plays a very important part in pregnancy, and occasionally a woman may deny her pregnancy, ignoring all the obvious signs of her condition, and refusing to seek any help or make any preparations. The pregnancy may be so successfully concealed, particularly if loose-fitting clothes are in vogue, that even her immediate family may be totally unaware of it until she is in labour or delivers.

CONFIRMATION OF PREGNANCY

The early signs and symptoms of pregnancy will make most women go to the general practitioner for confirmation.

Pregnancy tests   The general practitioner may perform a pregnancy test; these are now becoming more sophisticated and reliable, and nowadays some women will have done a test themselves at home. Pregnancy tests detect the presence of human chorionic gonadotrophin (HCG) in an early morning sample of urine.

Abdominal palpation   The pregnant uterus is palpable just above the pubic symphysis at about 12 weeks.

Vaginal examination   If the general practitioner performs a vaginal examination, there are certain physical changes in the vagina and cervix which are diagnostic of pregnancy. For example, the cervix becomes softer and the vulva and vaginal wall become purplish rather than pink as a result of venous engorgement.

Fetal movements   Women having a first baby usually feel the first fetal movements at around 20 weeks. (This is still referred to as 'quickening' from the old usage of the word 'quick' meaning alive.) Women having second or subsequent babies usually recognize fetal movements earlier, at around 16 weeks.

Few women are seeking confirmation of pregnancy before about 9–10 weeks' gestation, and most general practitioners would be reluctant to arrange antenatal care as early as this, since a certain number of pregnancies will end in spontaneous abortion before 12–14 weeks. The woman may still require advice and support for the discomforts of early pregnancy.

The care and advice offered to pregnant women is discussed in subsequent chapters.

FURTHER READING

LLEWELLYN JONES, (1982) *Fundamentals of Obstetrics and Gynaecology*, Vol. 1, 3rd edn. London: Faber & Faber.

SWEET, B. R. (1988) *Mayes' Midwifery—a Textbook for Midwives*, 11th edn. London: Baillière Tindall.

7

ANTENATAL CARE

PATTERNS OF ANTENATAL CARE

The vast majority of women in the UK will have their babies in hospital in the 1990s. Care was largely centralized in Consultant units in the middle and late 1980s, and GP units are decreasing in number. Home confinements are much less common than in the 1960s, though some women are wanting to have their babies at home, and the pendulum may well be set to swing. The centralizing of care, with the ideal of providing optimum facilities for the majority, while cutting down the expense of running small units, brings with it the threat of a vast, impersonal system. This has happened, and women have hated it.

Shared care

In order to provide the 'happy medium' in terms of care, the concept of shared care has evolved. This means that the woman has her pregnancy confirmed by the general practitioner, who refers her to a consultant obstetrician. The woman then 'books' at the consultant unit, where the rest of her antenatal care is planned. If she is fit and the pregnancy appears normal, she may only be asked to return to the hospital antenatal clinic once or twice more before she delivers.

The remainder of her care is then given in the community by her general practitioner and the community midwife. The system is flexible, to allow for instant referral to hospital should problems arise at any stage in the pregnancy. Her care may then be continued at the hospital, or back in the community.

In some inner-city or rural areas the consultant team may go out to a health centre or doctor's surgery to give antenatal care, so that mothers may come to familiar surroundings, and are more likely to attend. Ideally facilities are available at such clinics for almost all necessary investigations. This system has been introduced in a positive effort to reduce infant mortality and morbidity (which is higher in inner-city areas among the lower social classes) by good antenatal surveillance, health education and early detection of problems.

Consultant care

If a woman has medical or obstetric problems she may be advised to see the consultant obstetric team throughout her pregnancy. In some centres the obstetrician may run a 'medical clinic' together with a physician so that problems such as diabetes or cardiac disease may be managed efficiently.

Care in the community

While home confinements are not generally encouraged at present, the usual compromise is the 'domino' scheme (derived from the words domiciliary-in-and-out). Under the 'domino' system, the woman is cared for by the general practitioner and community midwife, and is taken into hospital for delivery. She and her baby are then taken home, usually no earlier than six hours following delivery. This means that she may be cared for at home during labour, and the midwife accompanies her to hospital at an appropriate time. All the consultant unit facilities are then available, with flexibility for transfer to consultant care should progress not be normal. Alternatively the woman may be delivered by her midwife and general practitioner in the GP unit.

Women are now being encouraged to return home as soon as they feel they want to do so, and many very new mothers and babies are being cared for by community midwives.

THE FIRST VISIT

The first visit to the antenatal clinic is an important one. First impressions will colour the woman's attitude to antenatal care, and if she is kept waiting for hours in a comfortless waiting area for a few apparently meaningless encounters with doctors and midwives, she will not be highly motivated to continue attending. Many women have felt like anonymous faces in a crowd, moving from one queue to the next. 'Patient' allocation rather than task allocation is as important in the antenatal clinic as it is in the wards.

The first visit is an occasion when a great deal of important advice is elicited and offered, and is ideally the start of a trusting relationship between the mother and the professionals.

Taking the history

The midwife will take the woman's history. This is a lengthy process because it is very comprehensive and should be conducted sensitively. Questions need to be asked carefully in order to elicit an accurate response, and phrased in such a way as to avoid patronizing the intelligent woman and mystifying the less intelligent.

Information will only be given if the woman feels relaxed, and confident in the questioner; some of the information she will give may be extremely personal and embarrassing to her. She may reveal facts from her past of which even her partner is ignorant. Confidentiality is therefore of paramount importance, and information must be recorded in her notes with care.

As the 'nursing process' approach is absorbed and developed by midwives, the first visit proves very useful as a basis for planning care with the woman. Unlike the nurse in the situation of acute illness, the midwife has a more predictable period of time in which to assist the woman to consider her care and her expectations, and to guide her in being realistic about these. This initial history taking may well be recorded in a 'care plan' type of format. Birth plans, not to be confused with care plans, are appearing more and more in women's notes. The 'birth plan' is a list of the woman's (or couple's) wishes regarding care before, during and after labour. It can provide an opportunity for sympathetic discussion and the start of a trusting relationship. The birth plan is usually completed later in the pregnancy when the couple have had the opportunity to explore options and thus to make informed choices.

The various aspects of history taking are summarized here, but different aspects will need to be expanded as necessary with different individuals.

Social history   This gives a picture of the woman as an individual, and provides a helpful indication of any problems she may have.

Personal details are recorded—name, address, age, marital status, occupation of the woman and her partner. Further questions may then be directed at finding out the kind of support the woman is likely to receive during and after her pregnancy, and whether or not she is adequately housed. Religion is noted, since this may give an indication of particular attitudes, beliefs or practices associated with childbirth, and also in general life-style, for example, dietary taboos. Nationality and language should also be recorded. A note as to how easy an immigrant woman finds it to communicate will be helpful, together with the name and telephone number of an interpreter where appropriate. Assumptions should not be made on the basis of marital status. The single woman may have planned her pregnancy; the married woman does not necessarily enjoy a supportive relationship.

Each woman's situation should be accepted sympathetically and without prejudice as far as possible. However, it should be remembered that the unsupported single girl from the lower social classes is at greater risk in terms of perinatal and maternal morbidity and mortality, and also in the longer term with regard to her general health, and that of her child.

Medical history A note is made of all previous hospital admissions, childhood illnesses, serious illnesses and medical problems. A note is made of any known allergy or sensitivity. From previous hospital admissions comes important information, such as details of any surgery, particularly on the genital tract, accidents involving bony injury to the pelvis, and any blood transfusions. Certain illnesses, such as acute rheumatism, may cause permanent damage, of which medical staff need to be aware.

Family history This includes questioning on prevalence within the families of both partners, where this information is known, of hypertension, diabetes, cardiac disease, multiple pregnancy, congenital abnormalities, and allergic conditions, such as asthma, eczema and hay fever.

Menstrual history Information regarding the regularity of the menstrual cycle, and duration of menstrual flow is helpful in indicating the likely reliability of the expected date of delivery. Any previous treatment for menstrual problems or infertility is noted.

Expected date of delivery (EDD)   The EDD is calculated by adding seven days to the date of the first day of the last menstrual period (LMP) and then adding nine months. For example:

LMP—4 April 1991: . . . EDD—11 January 1992
LMP—29 May 1991: . . . EDD—5 March 1992

It is common practice nowadays to confirm the EDD by the use of ultrasound scans. Accurate dating of the pregnancy is important if preterm labour should occur, or if there is any indication for inducing labour. However, the EDD itself is only an approximate guide as to when the baby is likely to be born, and delivery may occur within the 10 days beforehand or 10 days afterwards without being considered abnormal. Most women are aware of this, but may still be quite disappointed when 'The Day' comes and goes without a sign of labour.

Obstetric history   It is important to know how many pregnancies a woman has had, the length and outcome of each, and any problems which arose. Some complications are likely to recur, but the woman may be reassured that others probably will not. When obstetric history is recorded, a note is made of each baby's sex and weight, whether breast or artificially fed, and whether he or she is alive and well.

Physical examination

Part of this examination is carried out or supervised by the midwife, and is followed by a medical examination by the doctor.

1. Examination by the midwife

Height and weight   These are measured and recorded.

Urinalysis   Every woman is asked to bring a specimen of urine in a clean container each time she attends the antenatal clinic. The urine is tested to detect albumin and glucose, neither of which should normally be present. Glycosuria is not necessarily an abnormal finding, however, due to the lowered renal threshold in pregnancy (see Chapter 2). Repeated episodes of glycosuria require further investigation and continued surveillance. Albuminuria may be an indication of contamination of the sample by vaginal discharge, the presence of urinary tract infection, or more seriously, the development of pregnancy-induced hypertension or renal disease. A mid-stream specimen of urine is taken at booking in some centres, to examine the urine for asymptomatic urinary infection.

Blood pressure   The 'booking blood pressure' is regarded as an important baseline observation, and is referred to if the blood pressure rises during pregnancy. Anxiety and stress will tend to make the reading higher, as in any individual, but the effect of pregnancy initially is to lower the blood pressure. Thus a booking blood pressure of 90/60, for example, is quite normal.

Blood samples   Midwives commonly perform venepuncture, so this is listed here. Blood is taken to determine the woman's blood group, Rhesus factor, haemoglobin level, and rubella status (whether she is immune or susceptible to rubella) and the Wassermann–Kahn test for syphilis is performed. A test to measure alpha-fetoprotein (αFP) levels is usually offered in an attempt to detect neural tube defects (see page 91). Screening for such disorders as sickle cell anaemia, thalassaemia and hepatitis may be necessary for some women.

The breasts Although the doctor will usually examine the woman's breasts, he may prefer to leave more detailed advice on breast care to the midwife, and she too should look at the breasts, particularly the nipples.

2. *Examination by the doctor*

The doctor will examine the cardiovascular system, noting the blood pressure.

Examination of the abdomen The height of the fundus is noted at this stage; it should correspond with the gestation calculated by the EDD. A variation may suggest an inaccurate EDD or the possibility of a multiple pregnancy. The abdominal examination is usually performed in conjunction with an ultrasound scan.

Examination of the pelvis A vaginal examination may be carried out at the first visit, or a little later in pregnancy, unless there has been any suggestion of a threatened abortion, in which case it may not be done at all. The doctor is aiming to confirm the normality of the pelvic organs, to detect any pelvic masses, to assess the degree of uterine enlargement, and to confirm the pregnancy by noting certain changes in the vagina and cervix. He will also note whether or not the pelvis feels an adequate size.

The legs Probably the commonest finding here is varicose veins, especially in the multiparous woman. General advice is given, and support tights or stockings may be prescribed. Oedema should be noted; the examiner applies pressure over the tibia, to see if pitting occurs. Some ankle, pretibial and finger oedema in the last weeks of pregnancy, or in hot weather, is not abnormal. More excessive oedema, or swelling associated with rising blood pressure and albuminuria, can be a serious sign. Inequality of length, or muscle wasting, may be an indication of pelvic abnormality, whether congenital, or as a result of disease.

All the findings from the physical examination are recorded in the woman's notes, and also on the 'co-operation card' which she is encouraged to carry about with her at all times. The aim of this is to give a résumé of all her care so that whoever sees her at any stage will be adequately informed, and may write their own contribution in turn. In some centres women are being encouraged to keep their own notes, and to take them when visiting the hospital or health centre. This encourages women to take responsibility for their care and to know more about what is happening during their pregnancy, and provides a more detailed record for all concerned. It is hoped too that it will help break down some of the barriers between the public and the professionals.

SUBSEQUENT ANTENATAL VISITS

Following the initial visit, the woman will usually be invited to attend the antenatal clinic monthly until 28 weeks, then fortnightly until 36 weeks, and weekly until delivery. The venue for her continued care will be decided together with the woman as well as her general practitioner. Centralization of care may mean time-consuming, expensive bus journeys for some women, and this must be taken into consideration, particularly if she has to bring her other children.

At each visit certain investigations will be made:

Weight.
Blood pressure.
Urinalysis.
Physical examination including:
   abdominal palpation
   auscultation of the fetal heart
   inspection of the hands and feet for oedema.

Each visit should be as relaxed and informal as possible, with opportunity given for questions and discussion. Advice and general health education is offered whenever the opportunity arises.

ABDOMINAL EXAMINATION

The technique of abdominal examination is usually described under three headings—inspection, palpation and auscultation.

Inspection

This reveals the shape of the abdomen, which is usually described as ovoid or round. The firmer muscles of the primigravida give the neat ovoid shape, while the more lax muscles of the multigravida may make the abdomen appear larger and round. Size may be assessed visually and then checked on palpation. The presence of striae gravidarum (stretch marks) and any scars are noted. New striae are red in colour, those from a previous pregnancy or past obesity are silver-white. An unusually large abdomen with stretched, shiny skin might lead the examiner to suspect polyhydramnios—an excess of liquor, often an indication of fetal abnormality. Some students like to use the four S's to help them memorize the salient points when 'inspecting' the abdomen—Shape, Size, Striae, Scars.

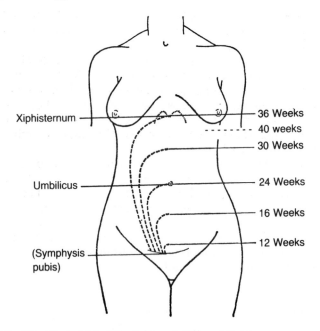

Xiphisternum —————

Umbilicus —————

(Symphysis
pubis) —————

————— 36 Weeks
- - - - - 40 weeks
————— 30 Weeks
————— 24 Weeks
————— 16 Weeks
————— 12 Weeks

Fig. 7.1 The height of the fundus at different stages.

Palpation

The size of the uterus should be appropriate to the
period of gestation throughout pregnancy, and any
deviation from normal is referred to the obstetrician
for further investigation. Although women vary in
their own stature as well as in the size of baby they
produce, fundal height can be closely related to the
period of gestation (Fig. 7.1).

The first stage in abdominal palpation is to feel for
the fundus of the uterus, and to relate it to one of
three landmarks—the woman's symphysis pubis, her
umbilicus or her xiphisternum. Some doctors have

returned to an old method, and measure the fundal height (though nowadays in centimetres), from fundus to symphysis pubis.

The examiner then elicits a series of specific details.

The *lie* of the fetus relates his spine or his 'long axis' to that of his mother. The lie may be longitudinal, oblique or tranverse (see Fig. 7.2). From about 34 weeks onwards the lie should be longitudinal. If the lie is longitudinal then the *presentation* must be either cephalic or breech.

Presentation is the next detail to be confirmed. Presentation may be defined simply as that part of the fetus lying lowest in the birth canal. It is described as vertex, face, brow, breech or shoulder (Fig. 7.3).

From presentation comes the *denominator* or *naming part*, and the denominator is related to the mother's pelvis in order to describe which way the fetus is facing, or the position.

The denominators are:

For a vertex presentation—the occiput.
For a face presentation—the mentum (the chin).
For a breech presentation—the sacrum.

A brow and a shoulder presentation are not given denominators since a fetus presenting in these two ways cannot be delivered vaginally, with the possible exception of a preterm baby presenting by the brow.

Having determined the presentation, the examiner goes on to try to determine the *position*. Relating the denominator to the mother's pelvis gives such terms as 'left occipito-anterior', (LOA), 'right occipito-posterior' (ROP), and 'left sacro-lateral' (LSL). The doctor or midwife feels for the fetal back which gives some indication of the position of the fetus. The position is determined more positively during labour by vaginal examination. Knowledge of the position may be academic during pregnancy, but is significant once labour

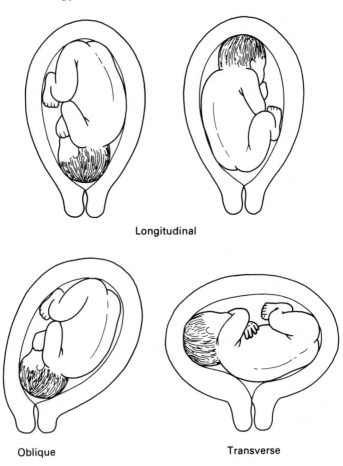

Longitudinal

Oblique   Transverse

Fig. 7.2   The lie of the fetus.

occurs, as it may have a bearing on the duration and outcome of labour, since some positions are more favourable than others (Fig. 7.4).

The *attitude* of the fetus relates his head and limbs

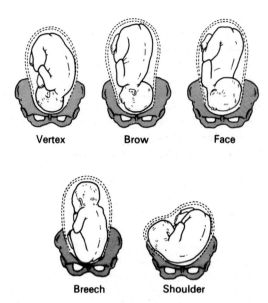

Vertex	Brow	Face

Breech	Shoulder

Fig. 7.3   The five types of presentation of the fetus.

to his body, and the attitude is described as flexed, deflexed (or 'poorly flexed') and extended. At the onset of labour the fetus is usually in an attitude of flexion.

Engagement is the term relating the fetal biparietal diameter to the maternal pelvic brim. Engagement usually occurs in a primigravida at 36 weeks, but in a multigravida may not occur until labour commences (Fig. 7.5). It is generally reckoned that if the fetal head will enter the pelvis it will pass through it successfully, though this may occasionally be untrue. It is therefore an important detail. Engagement of the fetal head is sometimes referred to colloquially as 'lightening', because of the sense of relief the woman feels when the pressure under the diaphragm lessens.

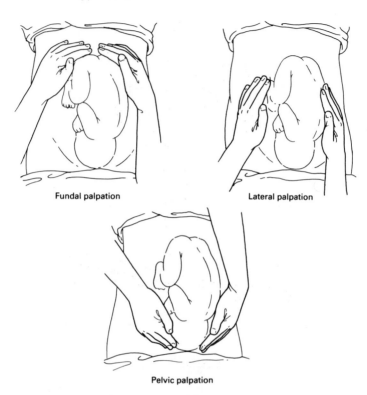

Fundal palpation

Lateral palpation

Pelvic palpation

Fig. 7.4   Types of palpation per abdomen

Auscultation

The fetal heart is heard through the abdominal wall, using a fetal stethoscope—the Pinard's stethoscope (Fig. 7.6). If the presentation is cephalic, the fetal heart is best heard through the lower part of the abdominal wall; if a breech, around the mother's umbilicus. Student midwives and medical students should aim to develop their skills with a Pinard's stethoscope, but

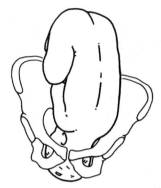

Fig. 7.5   Engagement of the fetal head.

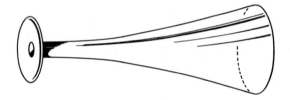

Fig. 7.6   Pinard's fetal stethoscope.

easier means exist, with ultrasound techniques—the Doppler, the Sonicaid and the cardiotocograph. Many of these devices are easily portable and are now widely used. The mother may hear the fetal heart easily when these are used.

ANTENATAL INVESTIGATIONS

The vast majority of women in the UK may now benefit from medical technology during their pregnancy if they so desire. However, medical advances bring certain ethical dilemmas, and screening for fetal abnormality must be accompanied by informative and sensitive counselling, since the logical progression from the discovery of fetal abnormality is to termination of the pregnancy in many people's minds. Some women may not accept this, however, and so they must be fully informed as to the implications of any investigations which may be offered to them.

Ultrasound scans

At the time of writing there is some unease, transmitted from the US via the media, as to the possibility of long-term ill-effects from the use of ultrasound scans. The 'take-up' rate of treatments and investigations will always be affected by such 'scares'. In the 1990s in the UK, this has not stopped obstetricians and radiologists regarding the ultrasound scan as an invaluable tool for diagnosis and surveillance. Scans are used in early pregnancy to:

Confirm pregnancy.
Confirm the EDD.
Diagnose multiple pregnancy.
Exclude fetal abnormality.

In later pregnancy they are used to:

Confirm the presentation of the fetus if there is doubt.
Detect retardation of normal growth.
Confirm the EDD.
Exclude certain fetal abnormalities.
Determine the position of the placenta.
Diagnose intrauterine death.

It is quite usual for an early scan to be performed as a routine, then any subsequent scans are performed only if there is some indication. If intrauterine growth retardation is suspected, serial scans may be performed in conjunction with placental function tests. The fetal skull, abdomen and limbs may be measured, and a regular series of such measurements gives a guide as to whether or not growth is proceeding normally.

Alpha-fetoprotein (αFP) measurements

This was mentioned under the heading of blood samples. Levels may be measured in maternal serum from 16 to 18 weeks. Raised levels may indicate multiple pregnancy, an error in EDD, or the presence of neural tube defect in the fetus. Recent research has suggested a link between a low reading and an increased incidence of Down's syndrome. Women with a low αFP result may therefore be offered amniocentesis, which must be done almost immediately.

Amniocentesis

In this investigation a sample of liquor amnii is taken from the uterus by passing a needle through the mother's abdomen under local anaesthetic. It does carry risks, including that of subsequent miscarriage, and so is done selectively following counselling of the couple. Down's syndrome may be diagnosed by examination of the liquor, and so amniocentesis is usually offered to the group at greatest risk, the older mother, though the age at which it is offered may vary. It is an example of an investigation which is not always offered if the woman would not wish to have her pregnancy terminated. The chromosomes may be examined for other hereditary abnormalities, and alpha-fetoprotein levels in the liquor may also be measured.

X-rays

Because of the possible long-term ill-effects of X-rays on the unborn child, and the probable relative safety of ultrasound scans (though this is still open to question) X-rays in pregnancy are used less frequently nowadays, apart from a special X-ray to measure the bony pelvis. This is called pelvimetry, and allows quite accurate assessment of pelvic size where diagnosis of possible cephalopelvic disproportion is important, in women of small stature, or those with a breech presentation.

Apart from this, women are advised to avoid having X-rays in pregnancy, particularly the early weeks, when possible. If X-rays of any other part of the body are necessary, the fetus is protected by means of a lead apron.

'Kick charts'

Research has shown that infrequent fetal movements are often associated with an unhealthy fetus. The mother is given a special chart, and asked to count the number of times she feels her baby move, say in the morning, and record it on the chart. Some doctors may ask her to record perhaps the first 10 movements from a given time. The mother is asked to telephone if she feels the baby moving less frequently, and she may then be asked to attend for a cardiotocography.

The cardiotocograph

A continuous recording of the fetal heart can be printed out on a graph by a special monitor. One transducer picks up the fetal heart beat, and the other records any fetal movements or uterine contractions, since the reaction of the fetal heart following either can be significant.

The use of fetal monitors is discussed in more detail in Chapter 11.

Placental function tests

Fetal well-being can be assessed by measuring levels of placental hormones in the mother. Placental deterioration occurs naturally if pregnancy continues much beyond term, and it is important to detect it early at whatever stage it occurs, or the fetus will become undernourished and then hypoxic. One single placental function test is unhelpful. A series of tests will be carried out over a period of time, and charted on a graph which shows normal ranges for the period of gestation.

There are two main tests.

Urinary oestriol   This is measured in the mother's urine.

Human placental lactogen (HPL)   This is measured in the mother's serum.

Chorionic villus biopsy (CVB)

Chorionic villus biopsy (CVB) or chorionic villus sampling (CVS) is a recently developed technique in which early placental, or chorionic, cells are taken for laboratory investigation, instead of liquor. The advantage of CVS is that it can be performed earlier than amniocentesis—at about 10 weeks, compared with about 16 weeks. It also leads to quicker diagnosis, so that earlier termination of pregnancy can be offered to the mother if there is any fetal abnormality. It is performed using ultrasound to locate the placenta, and the approach may be trans-cervical or trans-abdominal. There is a risk of subsequent spontaneous abortion, just as there is with amniocentesis, and it is only offered on a selective basis.

THE AIMS OF ANTENATAL CARE

In summary, the aims of antenatal care are:

To preserve, or even improve, the health of the mother.

To detect and treat early any abnormality of mother or baby.

To provide close surveillance for high risk groups including:

the very young (under 16 years old)
the older mother (over 35 years old)
the grande multipara
the lower social classes.

To improve general standards of health for the whole family by offering advice and health education.

To screen all women for certain conditions, for example rubella susceptibility and Rhesus incompatibility.

To screen high risk groups for certain conditions, for example Down's syndrome and hepatitis B.

To provide an informal, efficient service to encourage 100% take-up of antenatal care.

FURTHER READING

LLEWELLYN-JONES, D. (1982) *Fundamentals of Obstetrics and Gynaecology*, Vol. I, 3rd edn. London: Faber & Faber.

MATERNITY SERVICES ADVISORY COMMITTEE (1982) *Maternity Care in Action (Part I—Antenatal Care)*. London: HMSO.

MCCLURE BROWN, J. & DIXON, G. (1978) *Antenatal Care*. Edinburgh: Chuchill Livingstone.

ORR, J. (Ed.) (1987) *Women's Health in the Community* (Topics in Community Health Series). Chichester: John Wiley.

ROBINSON, S. & THOMSON, A. M. (Eds.) (1990) *Midwives, Research and Childbirth*. London: Chapman and Hall.

SAUNDERS, P. (1985) *Birth Wise* London: Sidgwick and Jackson.

SWEET, B. R. (1982) *Mayes' Midwifery—a Textbook for Midwives*, 10th edn. London: Baillière Tindall.

8

FURTHER PREPARATION FOR PARENTHOOD

ADVICE IN PREGNANCY

It is artificial to separate advice from a description of antenatal care (Chapter 7), although helpful in the interests of clarity, since advice and information are offered at all stages of care whenever the opportunity arises. If a trusting relationship exists between the pregnant woman and those offering antenatal care, she is likely to be very receptive to general advice and health education, if not for her own sake, for that of her unborn bay. Advice offered should always be realistic; for example, some women may not have the facilities or finance for vast improvements in diet, and the harassed mother of two or three preschool children probably cannot put her feet up during the day without some kind of outside help.

Advice and information are given during parentcraft classes as well as on a one-to-one basis at the antenatal clinic or in the home.

The areas covered will usually include the following.

Diet

A well-balanced diet is necessary if a healthy baby is to be born without robbing his mother of vital nutrients. Extra calcium and iron are needed; the fetus takes priority, and if his mother's intake of calcium is insufficient, her own dentition may suffer. The idea of 'eating for two' is no longer encouraged, but a good balance of protein foods, which can include the so-called second class proteins, with carbohydrate and fats, and plenty of fresh fruit, vegetables and salads, is advised. A pint of milk each day, or extra dairy products, such as cheese and yoghurt, should provide the extra calcium required.

Iron supplements are usually given only to women with a low haemoglobin.

The adjustment of diet to alleviate and then prevent constipation is discussed briefly on page 100.

Teeth

Dental decay occurs more readily in pregnancy because of the fetus's demands for calcium, and in an attempt to combat this, women in Britain are offered free basic dental care during pregnancy, and until the baby's first birthday.

Smoking and alcohol

There is now a much greater awareness and understanding of the risks from nicotine and alcohol to the unborn baby. Ideally women need to be made aware of these risks before they become pregnant, but some will need continued encouragement during the antenatal period to cut down on alcohol and nicotine consumption.

Other drugs

Ideally no drugs should be taken during pregnancy, but women should be encouraged to discuss routine medications with the general practitioner. Some prescriptions may need to be modified if a pregnancy is planned, and this is discussed in Chapter 4 in the section on preconceptual care. The critical period is the first weeks of pregnancy when the embryo is developing rapidly and vital systems are being formed. However, women may be reassured that the occasional use of paracetamol for a headache, for example, is unlikely to cause any problems.

Rest

Adequate rest is important, but many women in the tiring early stages of pregnancy may be working full-time as well as running a home; still others will be coping with lively, demanding toddlers. Women in advanced pregnancy may find it difficult to get comfortable and sleep at night and may need advice regarding the use of extra pillows. Swollen ankles may respond to sitting with the feet up and avoiding unnecessary standing, for example while ironing or preparing vegetables.

Exercise

Fresh air and exercise should be taken each day, and most sports can be continued, but pregnancy is not the time for unaccustomed, violent exercise. Exercises designed to improve the suppleness and tone of muscles used in labour are both popular and useful.

Sex

Women who have a tendency to miscarry or go into labour prematurely may be advised by the doctor not to have intercourse, though this need not preclude sexual activity. However, generally speaking, there needs to be no curtailment. Indeed, many women find they have increased libido and greater enjoyment during pregnancy. Experimentation with different positions may be necessary in the interests of comfort as pregnancy advances, and may be fun and very rewarding. Many men feel very tender towards their pregnant partner, and ideally pregnancy is a time of closeness and increased understanding and communication.

Hygiene

General standards of hygiene have improved over past decades, and most women have adequate facilities. However, some will still share a bathroom with other families, or feel unable to afford hot water. Advice in this area must be realistic. Perspiration and vaginal secretions increase during pregnancy, so a daily all-over wash is desirable. The use of vaginal deodorants is not necessary, and is discouraged.

The breasts

When the midwife sees the mother at the booking visit she will probably ask to look at her breasts. If the mother already feels sure that she wants to breast-feed, the midwife will examine her nipples. Normally the nipple protracts, that is, comes out, when the nipple is gently squeezed between the finger and thumb. Flat or inverted nipples may be improved by the use of 'Woolwich shells' which are worn inside the bra for a few hours daily. The earlier this treatment is started, the better the results, though some authorities doubt their usefulness.

If the woman is undecided as to how she will feed, this may give the midwife opportunity to offer some positive thoughts on the advantages of breast-feeding.

General advice includes keeping the breasts clean,

and the nipples free from encrusted colostrum. All women should be advised to wear a good bra which feels comfortable, and gives the breasts good support, with wide shoulder straps.

Financial benefits

Women may be very confused by the complexity of financial benefits, and the midwife should have a clear understanding of the system, so that she can help. Benefits are discussed in more detail in Chapter 19— 'Social Aspects'.

MINOR DISCOMFORTS IN PREGNANCY

Many of the minor discomforts in pregnany occur because of the effects of progesterone. Most do not need medical treatment, but may be eased by simple advice which the nurse can give, together with reassurance.

Morning sickness

Vomiting, or more commonly, nausea, is an unpleasant and frequent symptom in the first trimester of pregnancy. It is often alleviated by having a cup of tea and a plain biscuit before getting out of bed. If morning sickness persists beyond about the 14th week of pregnancy, or is excessive, it is known as hyperemesis gravidarum, and may require medical treatment in hospital.

Heartburn

This occurs because of the relative laxity of the oesophageal sphincter, and in later pregnancy because

of pressure from the gravid uterus. It is another unpleasant symptom, and may be relieved by simple
antacids if necessary. The woman may find it helpful
to sleep in a more upright position.

Constipation

This can usually be helped very considerably by adding
fibre to the diet; the use of unrefined 'wholefoods',
bran and plenty of fresh fruit, vegetables and salads,
together with an adequate fluid intake and sensible
exercise should help. Many women complain that their
iron supplement compounds the problem.

Frequency of micturition

This is caused by the growing uterus remaining anteverted in the pelvic cavity during the first trimester.
Once it becomes an abdominal organ, frequency of
micturition usually becomes less of a problem until the
final weeks of pregnancy, when there is generalized
pressure from the gravid uterus, and the presenting
part enters the pelvic brim.

Varicose veins and haemorrhoids

These occur as a result of progesterone effects on the
plain muscle of the vein walls causing laxity, and
relative inefficiency of valves, as well as raised intra-
abdominal pressure impeding venous return. Women
should be advised to avoid unnecessary standing, to
avoid pressure on the calves or restrictive clothing.
If support tights are prescribed, women should be
advised to put these on before getting off the bed in
the mornings. If haemorrhoids are a problem, dietary
advice to prevent constipation is helpful. Ointment or

suppositories may be prescribed to reduce pain and swelling. Women can be reassured that varicose veins and haemorrhoids occurring in pregnancy will usually resolve after delivery, though they will usually recur in subsequent pregnancies, and may then persist to some extent.

Cramp

This is thought to occur as a result of calcium deficiency, due to fetal demands on maternal stores, or to vitamin B deficiency.

Oedema

Ankle oedema, together with slight pretibial and finger oedema, is normal in the last few weeks of pregnancy, particularly in hot weather. The woman is advised to rest with her feet up as much as is practicable for her. A greater degree of oedema may be associated with 'pregnancy-induced hypertension' or with renal or cardiac disease.

Vaginal discharge

Cervical and vaginal secretions are increased in pregnancy, but the woman is referred to the doctor if her discharge is greenish, creamy, offensive or irritating.

Backache

This occurs as a result of laxity of the ligaments, particularly those in the pelvic joints. It may also be the result of poor posture, as the woman adopts an exaggerated lordosis in order to balance the extra weight from her pregnancy. Advice is given regarding good posture, and broad-heeled shoes are recommended for stability; advice is given regarding sitting with her back well supported, particularly if she has a sedentary job. Exercises may be suggested, in conjunction with the physiotherapist, to alleviate the backache, and to strengthen the back. Women should also be advised to lift carefully, with their backs straight, and to avoid stooping during housework, but to bend the knees, again keeping the back straight.

PARENTCRAFT AND RELAXATION CLASSES

Every pregnant woman should be offered the opportunity to attend these classes. The format may vary considerably between classes. One of the difficulties is that some women will want to know much more detail than others.

Traditionally the parentcraft part of the class has dealt with such matters as layette and the sterilizing of feeding equipment. Emphasis needs to be laid on basic principles and practical aspects. It is important nowadays to offer guidance as to which items of baby equipment are essential, and which may be improvised from existing household items. The wealth of sophisticated advertising with which she is bombarded can make shopping very difficult for the young mother.

Relaxation classes offer instruction in breathing and relaxation techniques, linking these with the processes occurring in labour. The National Childbirth Trust (NCT) offer more detailed courses of instruction, and these are very much geared to the couple. The personnel involved in parentcraft and relaxation teaching may vary. The midwife's training equips her to cover all the necessary ground, but often physiotherapists like to be involved in the relaxation part, and the health visitor has a useful contribution to make to the parentcraft part.

The surroundings should be as comfortable and pleasant as possible, the chairs set out in an informal fashion, and every opportunity given for audience participation in discussion and questions. A cup of tea gives an opportunity for informal chat, and prospective fathers should always be made to feel welcome. Too large a group will tend to inhibit the shy members, and may limit discussion. Too small a group may sometimes become rather intense, or members may feel uncomfortably conspicuous. A larger group may be halved, if two teachers are available, so that parentcraft and relaxation sessions may be run concurrently with each half, and then repeated for the remaining prospective parents. A crèche is a very helpful provision, if this can be arranged.

FURTHER READING

KITZINGER, S. (1977) *Education and Counselling for Childbirth*. London: Baillière Tindall.

NOBLE, E. (1980) *Essential Exercises for the Childbearing Year*. London: John Murray.

ROBINSON, S. & THOMSON, A. M. (Eds.) (1990) *Midwives, Research and Childbirth*, Vol. 2. London: Chapman and Hall.

SEDGBEER, S. & BUCHANAN, C. (1990) *The Single Parent's Survival Guide*. Wellingborough: Thorsons.

SWEET, B. R. (1988) *Mayes' Midwifery—a Textbook for Midwives*, 11th edn. London: Baillière Tindall.

VERNEY, T. (1982) *The Secret Life of the Unborn Child*. London: Sphere Books.

WILLIAMS, M. & BOOTH, D. (1985) *Antenatal Education*, 3rd edn. Edinburgh: Churchill Livingstone.

WORTHINGTON-ROBERTS, B. S., VERMEERSCH, & WILLIAMS (1985) *Nutrition in Pregnancy and Lactation*. Times Mirror/Mosby.

9

PROBLEMS IN EARLY PREGNANCY

ABORTION

Until 1990 UK law defined abortion as any interruption in pregnancy occurring before the 28th week. However, since babies born from 23 weeks now survive, there was much discussion over the appropriate gestational age which should be considered 'legally viable'. The 1990 Abortion Bill was very controversial; it allowed for termination of any pregnancy until 24 weeks' gestation given reasonable grounds, such as a threat to the mental or physical health of the mother. It also allowed for termination of the pregnancy at any stage if severe fetal handicap was diagnosed. At the time of writing the Abortion Bill has not been debated finally.

In common parlance abortion usually refers to an artificial means of interruption or terminating the pregnancy, and the term miscarriage is used to describe a naturally occurring event. In medical and nursing terms the word abortion covers both eventualities, but different types of abortion are described.

Spontaneous abortion

The symptom common to nearly every type is vaginal bleeding. An abnormal conceptus commonly aborts very early in the pregnancy, often at seven to eight weeks. At around 12–14 weeks the placental tissue should start to take over the progesterone production from the corpus luteum (see Chapter 2). If there is a hiatus and a fall in hormone levels an abortion is likely to result. Maternal infection may lead to abortion; uterine abnormality is another cause.

Sometimes there is slight bleeding as the tropho-blast embeds in the endometrium. This is known as implantation bleeding and occurs at around the time of the first missed period, so that it may confuse the dating of the pregnancy.

Threatened abortion Vaginal bleeding may be ac-companied by slight lower abdominal pain or back-ache. The placental tissue is only slightly separated from the uterine wall and bed-rest may preserve the pregnancy (Fig. 9.1). The woman will be anxious and often very upset, though this will depend on how welcome the pregnancy was. Even if the abortion is a relief the woman will experience emotional upheaval, and may need support and counselling at some stage.

Inevitable abortion The vaginal bleeding becomes heavier, uterine contractions are stronger, frequent

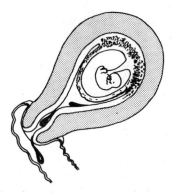

Fig. 9.1 **Threatened abortion.**

and regular, and the cervix dilates. In later weeks the membranes rupture. The abortion will progress to being complete or incomplete. The patient requires support and reassurance. Pain relief may be necessary and should be adequate for her needs. Temperature, pulse and blood pressure are monitored in order to detect any signs of infection or shock. Blood loss is estimated carefully and all pads and linen examined by an experienced eye for placental and fetal tissue. The doctor should be kept informed throughout.

Incomplete abortion   Evacuation of retained products of conception will be carried out under general anaesthesia. Any fetal or placental tissue remaining in the uterus will predispose to infection.

Complete abortion   The fetus and placenta appear complete.

Missed abortion   This is the one type of abortion where vaginal bleeding may not occur, although there

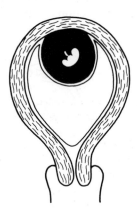

Fig. 9.2   Missed abortion (carneous mole) showing the ovum surrounded by a blood clot.

is often a brownish vaginal discharge. The embryo dies, and there is bleeding between the gestation sac and the uterine wall, but the uterine contents are not expelled immediately (Fig. 9.2). The symptoms of pregnancy gradually disappear, but the periods do not usually recommence until after expulsion or removal of the products of conception. Other names for this condition are carneous mole, blood mole or fleshy mole. The diagnosis is confirmed by ultrasound scan. The uterus normally expels the mole in due course, but the process may need to be induced as there is a risk of infection and of coagulation disorders.

Habitual abortion This term is used if a woman has three or more spontaneous abortions consecutively. The causes include uterine abnormality, low grade infection of the genital tract and cervical incompetence. Cervical incompetence may be the result of earlier terminations of pregnancy. Insertion of a Shirodkhar suture (cervical cerclage) may be effective.

Induced abortion

Induced abortion may be described as therapeutic or criminal abortion. Both carry immediate and long-term risks. The immediate risks are infection, haemorrhage and perforation of the uterus. Long-term risks include chronic infection which may lead to salpingitis and sterility, cervical incompetence and psychological problems.

In very simplified terms the Abortion Act of 1967 required that two registered medical practitioners should be agreed that continuing the pregnancy would put the health of the woman, her other children or the unborn baby at greater risk than terminating the pregnancy. The Act laid down conditions to try to safeguard women and prevent abuse of the provision. The next Abortion Act is likely to make similar provisos.

Therapeutic abortion   During the first three months of pregnancy therapeutic abortion is carried out by vacuum evacuation of the uterus. The patient is given a general anaesthetic. A wide bore hollow plastic curette attached to special suction equipment is introduced into the uterus under strict asepsis.

In the second trimester (third) of pregnancy termination is performed using prostaglandin, either by intra-amniotic instillation via the abdomen or by extra-amniotic instillation using a catheter passed through the vagina and cervix. Patients receiving prostaglandin may complain of nausea, diarrhoea or develop a pyrexia. Syntocinon (a synthetic oxytocin preparation) may be used in conjunction with the prostaglandin. If excessive stimulation of the uterus is given there is a risk of uterine rupture.

Another method is to withdraw some amniotic fluid and replace it with an equivalent amount of hypertonic saline. An intravenous infusion of Syntocinon is also commenced.

Before the prostaglandins came into use mid-trimester terminations were done by hysterotomy. This method is rarely used now because of the immediate and long-term risks to the mother.

Fig. 9.3 shows the possible outcomes of spontaneous and induced abortions.

Aspects of nursing care   With the advent of sophisticated means of prenatal diagnosis come difficult decisions for many women when they discover that they are carrying an abnormal fetus. When fetal movements are felt the pregnancy feels more 'real' and women begin to feel attached to the baby. Termination of pregnancy after this stage may therefore be more difficult. Deciding to terminate a pregnancy is

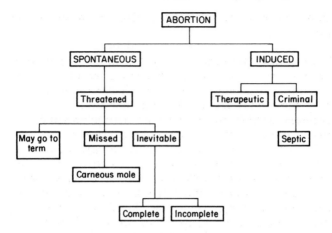

Fig. 9.3   The various possible outcomes of spontaneous and induced abortions.

rarely an easy decision and women need skilled, well-informed counselling beforehead. Some women may have few psychological sequelae at the time of termination, but experience a sense of sadness, loss and guilt in later years, often during subsequent pregnancies.

It is essential that the nurse should recognize the many conflicting emotions that women may feel. She may also need to face conflicting emotions within herself, and must be able to put aside her personal feelings and beliefs on order to give sympathetic, non-judgemental support. The woman who is aborting will value a supportive companion. She is likely to feel very isolated and vulnerable if she has not felt able to tell her family.

Physical care includes assessment of the woman's general condition and noting any change.

Blood loss is estimated and recorded, and the woman's temperature, pulse and blood pressure recorded as often as her condition warrants. Any rise in temperature is reported to the doctor so that impending infection may be diagnosed and treated promptly. Vulval hygiene should be given regularly, and sterile vulval pads used. Pain relief should be appropriate to individual needs, and should be given promptly. She may or may not wish to see the fetus, and her wishes should be respected and the situation handled sensitively. Following abortion she will continue to have some vaginal blood loss. This will become darker red and then brown and should diminish within two or three weeks. Any return to bright red loss or of an offensive smell should be reported to the doctor. Once the patient is able to get up she should be encouraged to use the shower or bidet at least twice daily.

Postoperative care following evacuation of retained products of conception or of vacuum termination is aimed at detecting any signs of infection, haemorrhage or uterine perforation as well as routine care of the patient who has undergone general anaesthesia.

Patients are discharged within hours of abortion if all is well. Women should be alerted to danger signs such as recurrence of bright red vaginal bleeding, abdominal cramps, general malaise or fever. Contraceptive advice should be offered, since ovulation may recur soon after the pregnancy has ended. The woman should be encouraged to see her general practitioner or gynaecologist for a follow-up visit.

Criminal abortion   This term is used when any attempt at procuring termination of the pregnancy is made outside the provisions of the Abortion Act. Such attempts are punishable in law, and the results may be disastrous. Haemorrhage, infection and perforation of the uterus are more likely than in skilled hands, and the woman may delay seeking medical help.

Septic abortion   This is a serious condition which may result from criminal abortion, or from infection following undetected retained products of conception. The severe infection may lead to septicaemia, renal failure and death. The infected uterus is more prone to rupture so that surgical intervention may be contra-indicated until the infection is cleared.

ECTOPIC PREGNANCY

Implantation of the fertilized ovum anywhere outside the uterine cavity is considered an ectopic pregnancy. Most frequently this occurs in the ampullary portion of the uterine tube (Fig. 9.4), but it may be ovarian, abdominal or cervical. Ectopic pregnancies are estimated as occurring once in every 250 pregnancies. Women with a history of one ectopic pregnancy have an increased risk of having a second one.

An ectopic pregnancy results when the passage of the zygote to the uterine cavity is impeded or slowed. Any blocking of the tube or reduction in tubal peristal-

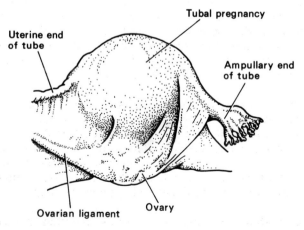

Fig. 9.4 **Tubal pregnancy.**

sis will achieve this. Former salpingitis, tumours and hormonal imbalances may all play a part.

As implantation occurs, the chorionic villi burrow into the thin tubal wall. Eventually, they burrow into a blood vessel, and bleeding occurs. If the bleeding is sufficient, the fetus dies. This is the fate of most. The abortus may be retained in the tube as a tubal mole or may be extruded through the end of the uterine tube as a tubal abortion. Occasionally, the trophoblast burrows through the wall of the tube and out into the peritoneal cavity. This is known as a ruptured tubal pregnancy (Fig. 9.5) and often occurs as the result of a pregnancy in the narrow isthmus of the tube. A secondary abdominal pregnancy may follow if the chorionic villi settle elsewhere in the abdominal cavity and begin to grow. This is rare.

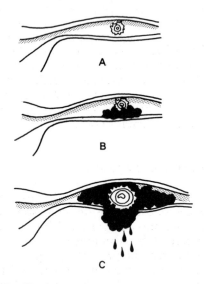

Fig. 9.5 A, Fertilized ovum in a uterine tube. B, Separation of the chorionic villi. C, Rupture of the tube.

Signs and symptoms

The accurate diagnosis of an existing ectopic pregnancy or a recently aborted ectopic pregnancy may be difficult. Fortunately, ultrasonography has simplified the task. These women may first be seen in the emergency department or in the clinic with a variety of symptoms.

The woman has a history of the early signs of pregnancy, including amenorrhoea usually of 6–19 weeks' duration. Soon after her first missed period she may have complaints of a localized pain on one side, due probably to the distension of the tube. Following that she may have sharper intermittent pain in the same area. This may be due to strong peristaltic waves of the tube attempting to pass the embryo or abortus along the tube. At some point the patient may experience a sharp, severe pain. This is probably synchronous with separation of the embryo and some haemorrhage. The sharp pain may be followed by generalized abdominal discomfort as blood spills into the abdomen. Referred shoulder pain may occur. Four or five days following this episode there is bleeding *per vaginam* due to falling hormone levels, which occur following the death of the fetus and cause the endometrium to regress and menstruation to occur.

Acute ruptured tubal pregnancy

Sometimes the patient reports no early symptoms but experiences one episode of acute abdominal pain shortly after her missed period. This acute pain is often accompanied by vomiting and fainting. Some vaginal bleeding may be present but appears too minimal to warrant the reaction of the patient. The patient may rapidly go into shock with a drop in blood pressure, rapid weak pulse, pallor, sweating, low tempera-

ture and cold extremities. The abdomen is distended
with blood and may be tight and tender to the touch.
A pelvic examination of the patient may be difficult
because of the exquisite tenderness. This is an emergency situation.

When the diagnosis of a tubal pregnancy is confirmed, a salpingectomy (removal of the uterine tube)
with the removal of the fetus is performed. This is
usually done within 24–48 hours of diagnosis unless the situation is acute, in which case it is done
immediately.

Ectopic pregnancies in other locations will be investigated in a similar fashion. Treatment is usually
surgical removal of the fetus. However, abdominal
pregnancies are carried to term and been delivered
by laparotomies.

HYDATIDIFORM MOLE

Hydatidiform mole is an abnormal development of
the chorionic villi of the conceptus. It begins to form
about the fifth week of embryonic life. The mole appears to occur when the fetal cardiovascular structure
fails to develop, but an intact trophoblast and a functioning maternal structure remain. As the fluid accumulates, the chorionic villi distend into small clear
vesicles, clinging to thin threads of connective tissue
in a grape-like pattern (Fig. 9.6). Few blood vessels
are present in the mass. Characteristically, there is no
fetus. Rarely, some mole-like degeneration may be
present on one part of an otherwise normal placenta.

The majority of women who have a molar pregnancy do not need to fear malignancy. Only 3–7%
of benign moles will proceed to malignancy.

The intermediate stages are characterized by an increased ability to invade uterine musculature and to

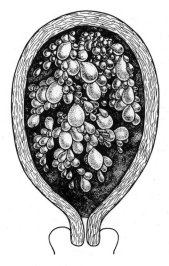

Fig. 9.6   A hydatidiform mole.

send bloodborne deposits of trophoblast cells throughout the body. However, in some cases, the host, or
pregnant woman, seems able to contain the spread
of the tumour and it disappears. The intermediate
stage is frequently not identified clinically, but is obvious only on pathological examinations of specimens
of tissue. This means that all moles must be treated as
potentially malignant until demonstrated otherwise.

Signs and symptoms

The patient exhibits the signs and symptoms of early
pregnancy. Vomiting may be more frequent. The uterus
is often much larger than expected for the weeks of
gestation. About the twelfth week, some vaginal bleeding may occur, and this is often the first sign of some

abnormality. No fetal movements are reported by the mother, and no fetal parts can be palpated. On palpation the uterus may have an elastic consistency. There is an increased incidence of pre-eclampsia. Urine tests for the quantity of chorionic gonadotrophins excreted show very high titres which persist and do not fall as is usual in a normal pregnancy. These high levels also stimulate the formation of theca lutein cysts in the ovary. The cysts regress following the abortion of the mole.

Treatment

Often the mole is partially aborted spontaneously. Haemorrhage may be acute. Oxytocics will be given to control the bleeding, and a careful and complete evacuation of the uterus will be done. Because of the danger of perforating the uterus in areas weakened by the erosion of the mole, a curette is not used. Instead, the cervix is dilated and suction equipment used to evacuate the uterine contents. Postoperatively the patient is observed for signs of haemorrhage.

Because of the possibility of a malignancy occurring, the patient receives close follow-up care during the next 12–18 months. The first signs of the recurrence of the mole or the development of a malignancy is a rising chorionic gonadotrophin level. Therefore, the urinary levels of gonadotrophin will be monitored at regular intervals. Amenorrhoea, metrorrhagia or persistent cystic ovaries may alert the gynaecologist to look for rising hormone levels. The patient is advised against pregnancy during this period, as early pregnancy also produces high chorionic gonadotrophin levels which could mask the signs. Cytotoxic drugs (such as methotrexate) are given in all intermediate cases, and may be given as prophylaxis to all women who have had a molar pregnancy.

CHORIONEPITHELIOMA (CHORIOCARCINOMA)

Chorionepithelioma is a malignant tumour of the embryonic chorion and is marked by invasion of the uterine musculature by malignant trophoblastic cells which have lost their original villous pattern. Destruction of uterine tissues with accompanying necrosis and haemorrhage is the result. The growth quickly metastasizes, and the most frequent site is the lung. The condition is extremely rare but because of its rapid advancement is considered to be one of the most malignant of all pelvic neoplasms. Death usually occurs within 12 months unless the patient receives early treatment. Fifty per cent of all cases of chorionepithelioma are preceded by a mole. The others are preceded by a normal pregnancy or abortion. Because of careful follow-up of patients who have had a molar pregnancy, the number of deaths from this disease have been reduced.

The chemotherapeutic agent methotrexate is the treatment of choice but may be combined with surgery. The drug is a folic acid antagonist and may be administered orally or parenterally for five consecutive days and then withdrawn for a week. The course may need to be repeated several times if chorionic gonadotrophin titres do not regress. Actinomycin D may also be used alone or in combination with methotrexate.

HYPEREMESIS GRAVIDARUM

Nausea and vomiting in early pregnancy is experienced by many pregnant women. After about 14 weeks' gestation persistent vomiting becomes an abnormality and requires further investigation. It is usual to admit the woman to hospital if there is ketonuria; if the condition progresses to this stage she will also be dehydrated.

Hyperemesis is exhausting and distressing. The woman may become very despondent, and will be anxious about the baby's well-being. She may usually be reassured once effective treatment has been established. An intravenous infusion of dextrose is commenced; serum electrolytes and urinary chlorides are estimated. The doctor may prescribe an anti-emetic and a hypnotic in extreme cases. There often appears to be an emotional element to this problem and many women who suffer from it have an anxious personality or may be under extreme stress.

DIABETES IN PREGNANCY

Research has shown that good diabetic control prior to conception greatly improves the outcome of pregnancy for both mother and baby. Diabetes can be very difficult to control during pregnancy as the mother's physiology undergoes such great changes. Ideally the mother is seen throughout pregnancy by her physician and her obstetrician, who work together. She will be booked for delivery in a consultant obstetric unit. She will need to test her blood glucose daily and test her urine for ketones. Her insulin requirements will normally be greater.

URINARY TRACT INFECTION

Urinary tract infection is more common in pregnancy because of the effect of progesterone, relaxing plain muscle in the ureters and bladder, causing stasis of urine. The commonest causative organism is *Escherichia coli*. Urinary infections in pregnancy may be asymptomatic apart from proteinuria on routine urinalysis at clinic visits, or the woman may complain of lower abdominal pain or backache, dysuria and frequency of micturition.

Infection may ascend to cause pyelonephritis, when the woman will complain of pain which may be in the loin on the affected side or may also radiate to the groin; she may have nausea and vomiting, with an elevated temperature and symptoms of cystitis. A mid-stream specimen of urine is obtained before a course of a broad-spectrum antibiotic is commenced. Nursing measures such as tepid sponging and fanning are employed to reduce the temperature since pyrexia and acute infection may lead to abortion or preterm labour.

The problem is likely to recur, sometimes following delivery, and the woman should be warned to seek medical advice immediately she is aware of any further symptoms.

FURTHER READING

FARRER, H. (1987) *Gynaecological Care*, 2nd edn. London: Churchill Livingstone.

GARDNER, R. F. R. (1972). *Abortion—the Personal Dilemma*. Exeter: Paternoster Press.

JONES, W. (1990) *Miscarriage—Overcoming the Physical and Emotional Trauma*. Wellingborough: Thorson's.

LLEWELLYN-JONES, D. (1972) *Fundamentals of Obstetrics and Gynaecology—Vol. 2—Gynaecology*. London: Faber & Faber.

WATSON, J. E. & ROYLE, J. R. (1987) *Watson's Medical-Surgical Nursing and Related Physiology*, 3rd edn. London: Baillière Tindall.

10

PROBLEMS IN LATER PREGNANCY

ANTEPARTUM HAEMORRHAGE

Antepartum haemorrhage is defined as bleeding from the genital tract after the 28th week of pregnancy.

There are two main causes, which will be described, but occasionally bleeding unrelated to the pregnancy may occur. The two conditions causing most cases of antepartum haemorrhage may also occur before 28 weeks (see Chapter 9), but the arbitrary division is made because of the greater likehood of fetal survival (see section on 'viability', page 70).

Placenta praevia

This term is used when the placenta is situated in the lower segment of the uterus. (Confusion may occur because early ultrasound scan reports may describe a placenta as 'low lying', but as the uterus enlarges, and the lower segment forms from about 30 weeks onwards, the placent may appear to 'migrate' away from the cervix.)

Placenta praevia is classified as type 1, 2, 3, or 4 (Fig. 10.1):

Type 1 lies within the lower part of the uterus, but does not reach the internal os.
Type 2 is situated with the placental edge just reaching the internal os.

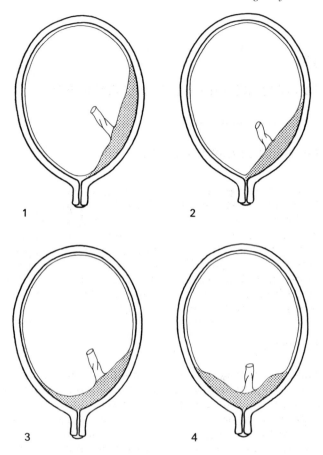

Fig. 10.1   Placenta praevia, types 1 to 4.

Type 3 is situated partially over the internal os.
Type 4 covers the internal os.

Placenta praevia causes painless bleeding, and careful observation in hospital is required. Vaginal delivery

is not safe, and may not be possible, if a type 3 or 4 placenta praevia is present, and caesarean section will be planned for about 38 weeks' gestation, provided no further significant bleeding occurs.

The presenting part is usually high, and the lie of the fetus may be unstable.

The first blood loss with a placenta praevia commonly occurs at about 30–32 weeks.

In any woman with an antepartum haemorrhage, the medical investigation and treatment is as follows:

Blood is taken for grouping and cross-matching. At least two units is usually requested.

If bleeding was severe, blood is sent for coagulation studies.

Rhesus negative mothers should have blood tests for Rhesus antibodies and the Kleihauer test. (Fetal cells may enter maternal circulation during placental bleeding.)

An intravenous infusion is commenced.

An ultrasound scan is performed in order to ascertain where the placenta is situated.

Examination in theatre may be planned at 38 weeks if there is doubt as to the diagnosis or degree of placenta praevia, or if ultrasound scanning facilities are not available. If this is done it may be with or without anaesthetic, but the theatre team will be standing by, ready to proceed to immediate caesarean section, since the examination can provoke further bleeding, which may be brisk.

Nursing needs

Reassurance and a full explanation must be given. The woman will feel much happier when she has heard the fetal heart. A cardiotocograph will be performed on admission.

Blood pressure and pulse will be recorded as necessary, and pads are inspected before disposal.

The woman will usually be allowed up for bath and toilet purposes if her general condition permits.

Constipation should be prevented by increasing fibre in the diet, and only if necessary by the use of gentle aperients.

Regular cardiotocographs will be performed.

The woman may be asked to maintain a 'kick chart'.

While bed-rest is prescribed, gentle leg exercises should be taught and encouraged, to minimize the risk of deep vein thrombosis.

Help may be needed with other children at home.

Boredom may be a problem, as the woman may be otherwise fit and well.

Placental abruption

This is the term used when a degree of placental separation occurs, and it is sometimes referred to as an accidental haemorrhage.

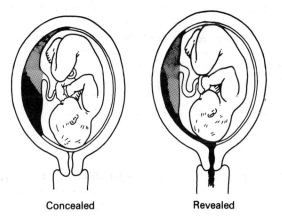

Concealed   Revealed

Fig. 10.2   Placental abruption.

It may be mild, moderate or severe; it may cause concealed or revealed bleeding, or both (Fig. 10.2). If the haemorrhage is completely or partially concealed, the woman will be suffering from a degree of shock greater than would be expected from the amount of blood seen. In severe placental abruption, the uterus is tender and tense, and is then described as 'woody'. Such bleeding may occur suddenly and dramatically, and the fetus frequently dies. The woman may be extremely ill, and the sudden hypovolaemia may cause coagulation defects, renal failure, and very rarely, Sheehan's syndrome.

Following a mild degree of placental abruption the woman may not be clinically shocked, and the cardiotocograph may appear normal.

Medical and nursing findings

History of severe abdominal pain, usually accompanied by vaginal bleeding.
Uterus is hard to touch, like wood, and tender.
Fetal parts are therefore difficult to palpate.
Shock may or may not occur.
Fetal heart may or may not be present.
Urinalysis may reveal proteinuria resulting from renal damage.

Medical investigations and treatment

These are as for placenta praevia; if pregnancy is to be allowed to continue regular placental function tests will be performed. Analgesia may be prescribed, to be given as necessary.

Nursing needs

These are as for placenta praevia, plus the following.

Analgesia must be given as necessary, if prescribed. Careful daily measuring of abdominal girth—an increase may suggest continued concealed bleeding. If caesarean section seems likely the patient may be starved, or allowed fluids only.

Incidental causes

Bleeding from the genital tract after 28 weeks' gestation, but unrelated to the pregnancy, is classified as incidental. It may arise from a cervical erosion or polyp, vaginitis, or very rarely from a carcinoma. Sometimes bleeding may not have been from the genital tract at all, but from haemorrhoids, for example.

HYPERTENSION IN PREGNANCY

When considering the pregnant woman with raised blood pressure, it is important to differentiate between hypertension caused by pregnancy, and pre-existing essential hypertension. Very rarely, another underlying cause, such as phaeochromocytoma, may exist.

Pre-eclampsia

By far the commonest cause of hypertension in pregnancy is pre-eclampsia, or as it is now increasingly known, pregnancy-induced hypertension. (Pre-eclamptic toxaemia, or PET, is an outmoded term, but refers to the same condition.)

There are three cardinal signs:

Raised blood pressure (definitions vary, but a common one is a persistent rise to 140/90 or over).
Oedema.
Proteinuria.

Pre-eclampsia may be defined as mild, moderate or severe. Its cause is as yet unknown; various theories remain unproven. It is commonly associated with multiple pregnancy, polyhydramnios, hydatidiform mole, and occurs more frequently in both the young teenager and the older mother.

Associated dangers include:

The development of eclampsia, when fits occur, and both mother and baby are severely at risk.
Placental abruption.
Renal damage.
Cerebral haemorrhage.

Medical and nursing findings

Raised blood pressure This is often defined as a persistent rise to 140/90 or more, but this will not necessarily be significant in women with essential hypertension. The 'booking blood pressure' is taken as a baseline, and any persistent rise of diastolic blood pressure to 20 or more above that at booking will be carefully monitored.

Oedema Almost all pregnant women have some oedema of feet, fingers and ankles at term, or in hot weather, but any further degree of oedema may be significant.

Proteinuria True proteinuria, which is not caused by urinary infection, contamination with liquor, vaginal discharge, or a dirty container, and can be demonstrated in a mid-stream specimen of urine, is a serious sign. It indicates that some degree of renal impairment or damage is occurring.

Symptoms Apart from oedema there are usually no symptoms, and the woman feels well.

Fetal growth   Once pre-eclampsia has been present for a while fetal growth may slow down because placental function is impaired.

Medical investigations and treatment

Investigation of hypertension to exclude other causes such as phaeochromocytoma.

Placental function tests—performed serially to detect placental deterioration early and so prevent fetal hypoxia.

Ultrasonography—performed serially alongside placental function tests to monitor fetal growth.

Rest is prescribed.

Anti-hypertensive drugs may be prescribed.

Diuretics may be prescribed.

The aim is to control the blood pressure and to deliver the baby at the optimum time for both mother and fetus if possible. Sometimes the baby may have to be delivered very prematurely in order to prevent any further deterioration in the mother's condition. The progress of pre-eclampsia is halted by delivering the baby.

Nursing needs

Regular and accurate recording of blood pressure.

Urinalysis—Esbach's test provides an assessment of proteinuria.

Careful observation of oedema.

Regular cardiotocography is performed to detect any early signs of fetal distress.

Encouragement to rest—the woman may be quite ill, but feel fit and well. She will need much support and encouragement.

Prompt detection and reporting of signs of fulminating pre-eclampsia is vital.

Strict fluid balance chart should be maintained.

Fulminating pre-eclampsia and eclampsia

Fulminating pre-eclampsia is the term used when pregnancy-induced hypertension or pre-eclampsia is about to reach a climax and cause eclampsia. It can be a very acute, rapidly progressing condition. It is serious.

Medical and nursing findings

Further rise in blood pressure—often sudden.
The woman may complain of:
frontal headache, often severe
visual disturbances
epigastric pain
general malaise
vomiting.
Oedema may increase.
Urinary output may fall.
Hyperreflexia is often present on neurological examination.

Medical treatment

Delivery of the baby is essential, and caesarean section is usually performed.
Stabilization of blood pressure by the use of anti-hypertensive drugs and sedation is attempted prior to delivery.
Blood is sent to the laboratory for clotting studies, as disseminated intravascular coagulation (DIC) may occur.

Nursing needs

Constant observation—an eclamptic fit may occur even after delivery, and the patient is usually kept sedated. A nurse must be with her constantly. Oxygen and suction should be at hand.

Careful monitoring of:

    blood pressure and pulse
    colour
    airway if under heavy sedation or unconscious
    urinary output
    proteinuria

Minimal disturbance—only essential care is carried out initially, and this must be planned so as to disturb the patient as little as possible. There should be a calm, peaceful atmosphere, but nursing in a darkened room is no longer carried out. Light must be sufficient to allow observation of colour.

If pregnancy-induced hypertension leads to maternal convulsions, the woman is said to be suffering from eclampsia. If she has not been delivered there is a real danger of fetal death. Fits are epileptiform, and the principles of management during a fit are to maintain a clear airway and to prevent injury.

General care is as for severe or fulminating preeclampsia. Maternal death may occur from asphyxia, cardiac failure or renal failure.

Essential hypertension

Essential hypertension may be present in the pregnant woman, just as in any of the population. It may be complicated by a superimposed pregnancy-induced hypertension. It is carefully monitored; antihypertensive therapy is usually continued during the pregnancy. If the woman was asymptomatic, the raised blood pressure may only have been detected at antenatal booking, and may therefore require investigation following delivery.

URINARY TRACT INFECTION

Urinary tract infections are more common in pregnancy, as the ureters become enlarged and tortuous because of the effect of progesterone on plain muscle, so that a degree of urinary stasis may occur. The commonest organism found is *Escherichia coli*.

Cystitis

Medical and nursing findings

Malaise.
Abdominal pain—lower abdominal pain may make the woman think she is an labour.
Urinary symptoms—the woman will usually complain of frequency of micturition, and burning pain on micturition.
The urine is opalescent, acid in reaction, and has a characteristic 'fishy' odour. Bacteriological examination reveals pus cells, red cells and organisms.

Medical investigation and treatment

Drug therapy—sulphonamides or nitrofurantoin may be prescribed. Potassium citrate mixture will reduce the dysuria by neutralising the acidity of the urine.
Analgesia—this will be prescribed as necessary.

Nursing needs

Fluid intake—the woman is encouraged to drink at least three litres daily.

Pyelonephritis

The woman is acutely ill.

Medical and nursing findings

Pain—radiating from loin to groin, often one-sided.
Pyrexia—often up to 39°C or 40°C, with rigors.
Malaise—headache, nausea and vomiting.
Urinary symptoms—cystitis is often present, with frequency of micturition and dysuria.
The urine—as in cystitis (see page 130).

Medical investigations and treatment

Bacteriological examination of the urine is carried out initially, after completion of antibiotic therapy, and again at the postnatal check.
Antibiotic therapy is usually instituted immediately, but culture and sensitivity results may indicate the need to change the antibiotic used. Antibiotics may be given intravenously.
Potassium citrate will render the urine alkaline and discourage further bacterial growth.
Analgesia is prescribed as appropriate.

Nursing needs

Nursing treatment of the pyrexia—tepid sponging and fanning are carried out as necessary.
Fluid intake is encouraged. An intravenous infusion may be commenced if the patient is very pyrexial and unwell. A fluid balance chart is maintained.

The incidence of preterm labour is increased when pyrexia occurs, so prompt and appropriate treatment is important for this reason, as well as to preserve good renal function in the future.

BLOOD DISORDERS

Anaemia

The commonest blood disorder seen in pregnancy is iron deficiency anaemia. Opinions vary as to the need for iron supplements in pregnancy, but many obstetricians now give these only if the haemoglobin is low. Folic acid is often given with the iron.

If the anaemia is severe, or is detected late in pregnancy, it may be necessary to give parenteral iron. Intramuscular injections of iron are painful and unpleasant, and the course takes several days to complete, depending on the total dose required.

Intravenous administration of iron is relatively quick and effective, but adverse reactions are not uncommon, and the woman must be observed carefully during the treatment.

Sickle cell anaemia

This is a haemolytic anaemia seen in women from Central and West Africa and parts of Asia. It is a hereditary condition, and many women have a heterozygous form, known as a 'sickle cell trait'. Those women having the homozygous form have sickle cell disease; their red cells have the characteristic sickle shape, and are particularly prone to haemolysis. The baby will need careful follow-up too; 'sickling' does not occur in the neonatal period.

Thalassaemia

This is another form of hereditary haemolytic anaemia, seen most commonly in women from the Mediterranean countries.

Rhesus incompatibility

The Rhesus negative mother with a Rhesus positive fetus is at risk of forming antibodies following delivery. Although fetal and maternal blood do not mix, there may be 'spill-over' of fetal cells into the maternal circulation when the placenta separates. Antibodies are produced, and in a subsequent pregnancy these may cross the placenta, and with a Rhesus positive fetus cause haemolysis of fetal red cells. In order to prevent this, Rhesus negative women are given an intramuscular dose of anti-D immunoglobulin following delivery. Other women at risk of 'spill-over' of fetal cells are those who have had an abortion or a placental abruption; occasionally 'spill-over' may occur following amniocentesis (see page 91). Maternal blood is examined for the presence of fetal cells, using the Kleihauer test. In some centres the anti-D immunoglobulin is given to all Rhesus negative women without waiting for the results of the Kleihauer test. Maternal blood is tested for Rhesus antibodies throughout pregnancy.

PRETERM LABOUR

If labour commences at any stage before about 36 weeks' gestation, it is important that the woman is cared for where there are facilities available for a preterm baby. It is always preferable to transfer a preterm baby *in utero* to a suitable centre for delivery.

The whole question of attempting to inhibit preterm labour is a vexed one, to which there is no easy answer, and on which doctors will not always agree. Factors taken into consideration include:

The period of gestation.
Whether or not labour is truly established.

Whether membranes are intact or ruptured.
Obstetric history—of both present and previous pregnancies.

Inhibition of preterm labour involves the use of a beta receptor stimulant drug, such as ritodrine hydrochloride, salbutamol or isoxsuprine hydrochloride (Duvadilan), given in carefully controlled dosages by intravenous infusion. These drugs cause unpleasant side-effects, and there will usually be a maternal and fetal tachycardia. The woman will often complain of palpitations, sweating, nausea and vomiting, and feeling flushed.

Nursing needs

Full explanation and reassurance.
Help with basic hygiene and comfort.
Support and encouragement during unpleasant treatment.
Careful observation of maternal and fetal condition, keeping medical staff fully informed of all developments.

CEPHALOPELVIC DISPROPORTION

As its name suggests, this occurs when the fetal head appears too large to pass through the pelvis. This may be because the fetus is unusually large, or is abnormal, or because the pelvis is unusually small, or is abnormal.

In the primigravida, the fetal head usually engages at about 36 weeks. If the head remains high an X-ray pelvimetry is performed, to assess pelvic measurements, and to determine the type of pelvis (see page 32).

In the multigravida, the likelihood of a successful vaginal delivery can be assessed largely on previous obstetric history, together with progress in the present pregnancy.

If there is some suggestion of cephalopelvic disproportion, the obstetrician may decide to allow the woman a short 'trial of labour'. This involves giving her a previously decided period of time in established labour, culminating in caesarean section if she does not progress as anticipated. Such a decision should be discussed with the woman and her partner, as well as with the midwife, so that all concerned can reach a reasoned decision with which everyone is happy. Progress is carefully monitored, as well as maternal and fetal condition, and the situation is reassessed at regular intervals.

It is not considered good obstetric practice nowadays to allow labour to proceed without good progress, nor for difficult or potentially difficult forceps deliveries to be performed. Caesarean section is therefore performed more readily than even 10 years ago, in the interests of both maternal and fetal well-being.

MALPOSITION

The optimum position for the fetal head is occipito-anterior, well flexed, so that the vertex is presenting. Any other position is known as a malposition, and a larger diameter of the fetal head then has to pass through the pelvis, so that delay, difficulty and trauma to mother or baby are all more likely.

The commonest malposition is an occipito-posterior position (Fig. 10.3). It often occurs in primigravidae, and tends to prolong labour, often causing distressing backache, which is difficult to alleviate satisfactorily.

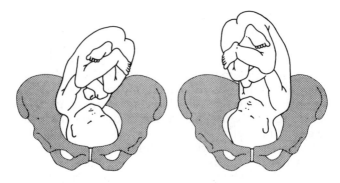

Fig. 10.3   Right and left occipito-posterior positions.

MALPRESENTATION

At term the fetus is normally presenting by the vertex. Presentation by any other part is known as malpresentation. These are:

    breech
    face
    brow
    shoulder

In a breech presentation the buttocks enter the pelvic brim. Breech presentations (Fig. 10.4) may be classified as follows.

Flexed breech   The legs are flexed in the normal 'fetal position'.

Extended or frank breech   The legs are extended or straight, so that they are splinted against the trunk.

Footling breech   One or both feet present before the buttocks.

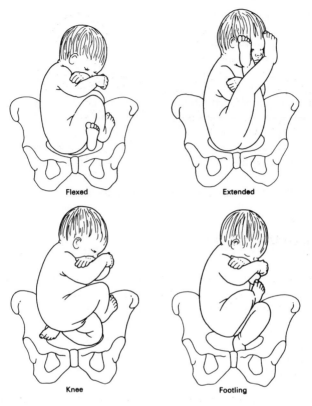

Fig. 10.4 Types of breech presentations.

Kneeling breech This is uncommon; one or both knees present before the buttocks.

Breech presentation is common in preterm labour, since the fetus usually turns to present by the vertex by about 34 weeks' gestation. It is also common in a twin pregnancy, or if there is oligohydramnios (scant liquor), so restricting fetal movement in the uterus, or polyhydramnios (excessive liquor) allowing free fetal movement; a hydrocephalic fetus will commonly present by the breech.

Because of the risks to the fetus, a primigravida with a breech presentation will often be delivered by elective caesarean section. X-ray pelvimetry will often be performed. The fetal head is its largest part, and great care must be taken to avoid the situation where the entire baby is delivered and then the head is found to be too large. In a normal vertex delivery, the fetal head moulds throughout labour, so that the pelvis can accommodate it; in a breech presentation this does not occur. Control of the head is very important, so as to prevent injury to the baby, and the head is usually delivered by forceps for this reason.

Face presentation is not common; it occurs in approximately 1:500 deliveries. A face presentation may be delivered vaginally in many cases. The baby's face remains bruised and oedematous for a few days after birth.

A brow presentation is not normally delivered vaginally, except possibly with a small, preterm baby. Once diagnosed, immediate caesarean section is usually performed.

A shoulder presentation cannot be delivered vaginally.

MULTIPLE PREGNANCY

Twin pregnancy arises either from the fertilization of more than one ovum, giving dizygotic or binovular twins, or from the splitting of a fertilized ovum (the zygote), to give monozygotic (or uniovular) twins. In a multiple pregnancy with more than two fetuses, both phenomena may be seen.

Multiple pregnancy is often diagnosed early, with

the use of ultrasound scans to confirm pregnancy and gestation. However, it may be suspected clinically in the woman who is larger than expected from the date of her last menstrual period, who is suffering from exaggerated 'minor disorders' of pregnancy, or who has unusually high alpha-fetoprotein levels.

Complications include:

Preterm labour.
Exaggerated 'minor discomforts'.
Increased incidence of pre-eclampsia.
Increased incidence of anaemia.
Extreme discomfort and increased pressure symptoms towards term.

Twins may usually be delivered vaginally, unless there is any other complicating factor. More than two fetuses are usually delivered by caesarean section.

PROBLEMS IN THE FETUS

Intrauterine growth retardation

When the fetus is found to be smaller than expected for the period of gestation, this usually indicates some degree of placental insufficiency, and less often, some fetal abnormality. The placenta normally starts to function less efficiently at some point after about 41 weeks' gestation. In pregnancy-induced hypertension, or in women who smoke heavily, the placenta may be unhealthy. The risk then is of fetal hypoxia, as well as retarded growth, with the possibility of intrauterine brain damage. Such a baby is not well equipped to withstand the stress of labour.

It is therefore very important to detect intrauterine growth retardation (often abbreviated to IUGR) early, and monitor fetal well-being very carefully.

The following investigations are described more fully in Chapter 7:

ultrasound scans
placental function tests
fetal monitoring
kick charts

If placental function appears to be deteriorating, delivery may have to be expedited, and caesarean section may sometimes be necessary.

FURTHER READING

BOTTING, B., MCFARLANE, A., & PRICE F. (1990) *Three, Four and More, A Study of Triplet and Higher Order Births*. London: HMSO.
DONALD, I. (1979) *Practical Obstetric Problems*. London: Lloyd-Luke Medical Books.
LLEWELLYN-JONES, D. (1982) *Fundamentals of Obstetrics and Gynaecology*, Vol. I, 3rd edn. London: Faber & Faber.
SWEET, B. R. (1988) *Mayes' Midwifery—a Textbook for Midwives*, 11th edn. London: Baillière Tindall.

11

NORMAL LABOUR

Labour is the physiological process whereby the fetus is expelled from the uterus. Labour is described in three stages, defined as follows.

First stage This commences with regular contractions, usually painful, associated with dilatation of the cervix, and ends at full dilatation of the cervix.

Second stage This commences with full dilatation of the cervix, and ends with the complete expulsion of the fetus.

Third stage This commences with complete expulsion of the fetus, and ends with complete expulsion of the placenta and membranes.

It is very important to define the onset of labour correctly. The uterus contracts during pregnancy; these contractions are sometimes described as 'warm up' or 'practice' contractions. They are called Braxton Hicks contractions, and do not cause appreciable dilatation of the cervix. They are irregular, and are said to be painless; some women would disagree with this! However, some women are barely aware of them.

Recognition of labour The onset of labour for some women is heralded by the rupturing of the membranes. Women should report this to the hospital, even if contractions do not commence. There is some risk of infection once the membranes have ruptured, and if the pregnancy has gone full term, labour will be expedited, perhaps after 24 hours.

Some women will have a 'show' as labour commences, others will not. The 'show' is a mucoid vaginal loss, usually streaked with blood which may be dark or bright. The mucus originates from the cervical canal, and is expelled as cervical effacement and dilatation occur.

Although it is impossible to tell women exactly what to expect, it is usual to advise them to go to the hospital when their contractions are occurring regularly, about every five minutes.

Every woman's experience of labour is different, and it is therefore wrong to be dogmatic, but it is usual to describe a latent and an active phase in both the first and second stages of labour.

A primigravid and a multigravid labour are quite different.

The latent phase of the first stage is the period of time during which the uterus contracts regularly (though perhaps not very frequently) and probably painfully, though this varies. These contractions achieve effacement of the cervix, and dilatation to 3–4 cm.

The active phase then follows, and should achieve full dilatation of the cervix at a rate of about one centimetre per hour in a primigravida. It is this period of time which is subject to close scrutiny in 'active management of labour', and most obstetricians would prefer it not to be prolonged. This is because the active phase is the time when the fetus is more at risk, and it is generally felt that a long labour is likely to exhaust both mother and baby.

SOME DEFINITIONS

Effacement of the cervix   This is the process whereby the contracting uterus causes the internal os to open,

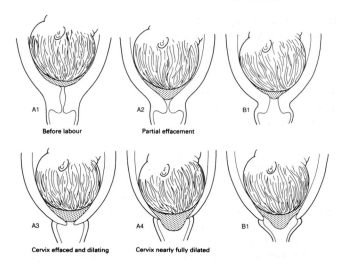

Fig. 11.1 Effacement and dilatation of the cervix: A, in a primigravida; B, occurring simultaneously in a multigravida.

the cervical canal shortens and disappears, and then the external os dilates (Fig. 11.1). In a multigravida the external os may be open, but the cervical canal may still be felt on vaginal examination.

Active management of labour In an attempt to reduce perinatal mortality, obstetricians have become much more involved in the care of women in labour over the past two decades. There is no doubt that a long labour is detrimental to both mother and baby, but the difficulty lies in finding the right balance. However, active management is aimed at reducing the length of labour by means of rupturing the membranes and giving oxytocin by intravenous infusion, in order to achieve steady dilatation of the cervix.

Active birth This should not be confused with the previous definition! Because women have resented being 'managed' (largely by male obstetricians) a vocal minority in recent years have demanded more say in their care, greater flexibility in the approach of all professionals, and a return to the natural physiological processes. The active birth lobby have been greatly influenced by the practice and writings of Michel Odent, in France. In an active birth the woman and her partner ideally work closely with the midwife, planning beforehand what they wish and do not wish. They will expect to move around during labour, being upright as much as possible, and to deliver in a position they find comfortable when the time comes, perhaps squatting or kneeling. They will want no medical intervention if possible. This whole concept calls for flexibility, in the woman as well as her attendants, and she must be encouraged to be realistic about labour, which is aptly named!

CARE IN LABOUR

The challenge for the midwife working in the labour ward is in getting to know a woman, gaining her trust and confidence, and caring for her during one of the most important experiences in her life. Now that women expect to survive childbirth and to have a baby who is in optimum condition, and not just alive, they are placing much more emphasis on the emotional experience. The quality of care a midwife gives is one of the most important factors in this. The student nurse, working in the labour ward, in great fear and trepidation maybe, is in a position to enhance this care by her continual presence and involvement, as the midwife may have other women to care for. Ideally, of course, the midwife should be able to meet the woman beforehand and get to know her before she goes into labour, and then should care for her throughout, and some schemes have been set up to try and achieve this. In the 'team approach' a group of mid-wives will care for the woman during her pregnancy, and one of the team will deliver her. It is very difficult to prepare women for labour, since it will be different for all of them. Because it is such a major life event, involving strange faces in a strange place, and much that is unknown, many women will be very apprehensive. A large component of the care given is therefore emotional support—reassurance, encouragement, keeping the woman and her partner informed of progress and prognosis.

It is the situation where the student nurse will utilize her nursing skills most in obstetrics.

The first stage

Nursing needs

Hygiene and comfort Many women will be up and about during the first stage, and may take a bath or shower as required. A warm bath may be very soothing as well as refreshing. If the woman is in bed, a fan, iced water to suck, frequent mouthwashes and a damp, cool flannel, are all appreciated. The partner may be encouraged to help with this kind of comfort; some may feel awkward in this situation, and are relieved to be given a job to do.

Position This is an important aspect of comfort; the woman may not be able to find a comfortable position, but the midwife can often make helpful suggestions. It is now common to find rocking chairs, reclining chairs and bean bags in the labour room, and these, together with plenty of pillows, should be used imaginatively. It is important, if the woman is lying down, that she should not be completely flat. This is because the weight of the gravid uterus, pressing on the vena cava, may cause aorto-caval occlusion, leading to reduced cardiac output, and then reduced placental blood-flow. A small rubber wedge, or a folded blanket under the mattress, is usually sufficient to prevent this.

Bladder care   As the fetal head descends, it becomes increasingly difficult for the woman to pass urine. She may lose the sensation of a full bladder. A full bladder may impede the progress of labour, and is liable to be damaged, so it is important to encourage micturition every two hours, and to keep a careful record. Only if necessary will the midwife pass a catheter prior to vaginal examination.

Bowels   The days of routine enemata are largely past. Most women report frequent, loose bowel movements prior to labour, but suppositories are given if necessary, since a full rectum will slow down descent of the head, and may cause the woman great embarrassment at delivery or in retrospect.

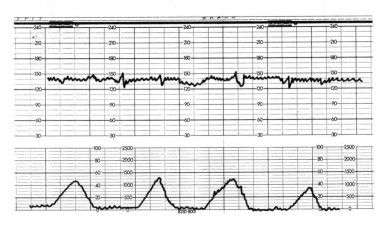

Fig. 11.2   **A normal cardiotocograph showing the variable heart rate of the healthy fetus. The upper tracing is the fetal heart rate, while the lower line shows the uterine contractions.**

Diet   It is not usual to allow women in labour to eat,
though a few will complain of being ravenously hungry
in the early stages. The stomach usually remains full,
and many women vomit in labour. The full stomach
is a potential hazard if a general anaesthetic should
be required at any stage. Some women may wish to
suck glucose sweets, and the midwife will allow this
at her discretion. Low residue foods, such as plain
biscuits and tea are also permissible if the woman
wishes.

Pain relief   The midwife, in caring for women in normal labour, may give appropriate analgesia within
certain parameters.

Fetal monitoring

Cardiotocography (CTG) is one of the technical advances which were hailed with great delight, but is
now subject to review. For a time after its introduction
women in labour were monitored continuously, but
the problem with this is that they cannot be fully ambulant, and many women therefore dislike it. There is
a small, portable system available, called telemetry, but
it too has its disadvantages.
    The cardiotocograph (Fig. 11.2) is a device designed
to give a continuous read-out, in graph form, of the
fetal heart beat on one line, and of uterine contractions and fetal movements on the other.

External fetal monitoring   This involves the use of
two external transducers, strapped to the mother's
abdomen using elastic belts. Some women find this
uncomfortable in labour.

Internal fetal monitoring   This involves rupturing
the membranes, if they are still intact, and applying

a fetal scalp electrode to the baby's head. This device is attached by means of a fine sprung wire, which just pierces the skin. It is also possible to measure intra-uterine pressure, and therefore assess the strength of contractions, with an intrauterine catheter, but these are no longer widely used.

Interpretation   The midwife caring for a woman in normal labour must be able to recognize an abnormal or suspect cardiotocograph, and take prompt, appropriate action.

Fetal heart rate patterns   The normal rate is 120–160. The rate should vary—'beat to beat variability', and the fetal heart should respond to the stress of uterine contractions, which is why they are recorded in tandem.

Type I dips are defined as a slowing of the fetal heart with a contraction, with a return to normal by the end of the contraction. They are interpreted alongside factors such as dilatation of the cervix, length of labour and colour of the liquor.

Type II dips occur later in relation to the contraction, and may be a sign of fetal hypoxia. The obstetrician is informed, and a sample of fetal blood from the scalp is usually taken (fetal blood sampling or FBS), and its pH measured to detect fetal hypoxia.

The partogram

The partogram is an extremely useful document. It provides a graphic display of the progress of labour, together with the midwife's observations, fluid intake and output, and any analgesia or other drugs given (Fig. 11.3).

It was introduced at the time when active management of labour became popular, and the idea was that an 'action line' should be drawn at the time when

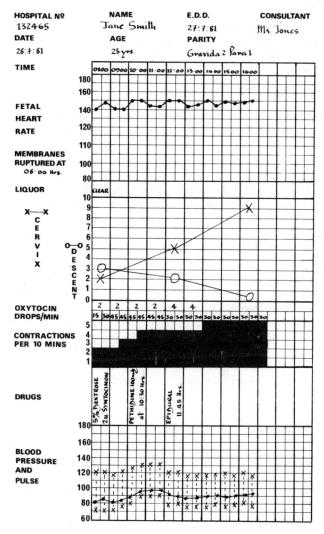

Fig. 11.3   A partogram.

delivery should occur, and that if spontaneous delivery did not appear to be imminent when this time came, caesarean section should be performed.

The midwife's observations

The midwife makes certain observations throughout labour. She assesses the progress of labour by noting:

Contractions—the length, strength and frequency.
Descent of the presenting part by abdominal palpation and also by vaginal examination.
Cervical effacement and dilatation by vaginal examination.

She also records:

Blood pressure.
Pulse.
Temperature.
Fluid intake and output.
Urinalysis—performed each time the woman passes urine, looking for ketones and albuminuria.
All analgesia given.
Any other drugs given.

Care in the second stage of labour

There are certain clinical signs indicative of the second stage of labour.

A heavy 'show' is often seen.
'Bulging' of the perineum.
Gaping of the anus, often with some faeces being passed.
The vertex may be visible.

The mother may say that she wants to push, or she may just grunt or push involuntarily.

The latent phase of the second stage is described as the time from full dilatation of the cervix to descent of the head onto the perineum, so that the vertex is visible, and the woman has an overwhelming urge to bear down. The active phase then commences, and the woman is encouraged to push. For many women these two phases are not clearly defined, but it can be useful to make this distinction if a woman has had epidural analgesia, for example, and has no urge to bear down. If the head is allowed to descend spont-aneously, she is much less likely to exhaust herself, and is then able to push effectively. The risk of hy-poxia to the fetus is no greater in the second stage before pushing commences than it was in the first stage, and it is not the length of the second stage itself which is seen as most important, but the duration of active pushing.

Some women will request dimmed lighting for de-livery, but it is still possible to direct a good light on the perineum.

Delivery is conducted using aseptic technique, with sterile towels and instruments. If the woman is kneel-ing or squatting, clean sheets may be placed on a mat-tress on the floor, and the delivery pack placed on another clean sheet.

Normal delivery As the vertex advances, the mid-wife may control its advance, and encourage flexion (so that the smallest diameter of the head distends the perineum) with one hand, or it may be sufficient to instruct the mother how to breathe. The midwife watches the perineum closely; it is designed to stretch to accommodate a baby, but if it shows signs of in-adequate stretching, she will infiltrate with local an-aesthetic solution prior to performing an episiotomy.

The episiotomy is performed at the height of a contraction, as the perineum is fully distended and thinned, using special scissors.

'Crowning' is the term used to describe the delivery of the biparietal diameter, the widest part of a well-flexed head. Once the head is delivered, the midwife feels for cord around the baby's neck. (If tight, it will be clamped and cut, otherwise it may be slipped over the head, or over the shoulders as the body is born.)

With the next contraction, the mother is encouraged to give a long, steady push, and the body will be born. The second stage is then complete.

The baby is usually delivered onto the mother's abdomen, so that she may see and touch him immediately. He is dried thoroughly, to prevent chilling, and then covered with warmed blankets.

At birth he will be an alarming shade of purple, and the new parents may be anxious, as they may be if he does not immediately cry. However, a baby who has had a calm, peaceful delivery may not cry; as long as he breathes spontaneously and becomes pink, the parents may be reassured. His hands and feet may remain blue for some time after birth. If the baby has mucus in his air passages, and does not clear it himself, the midwife may gently suck out his mouth and nostrils.

Resuscitation of the baby Some babies may need more active resuscitation, and every midwife is trained to do this. A 'Resuscitaire' should be readily available; this piece of equipment provides a safe, convenient working surface with an overhead light and heater, to prevent chilling, together with suction apparatus and a means of giving oxygen (Fig. 11.4). Easily accessible drawers contain all that is required to intubate the baby. If any problem is anticipated, for example, with an abnormal delivery, a preterm baby, or severe fetal distress, the paediatrician will usually be present to receive the baby.

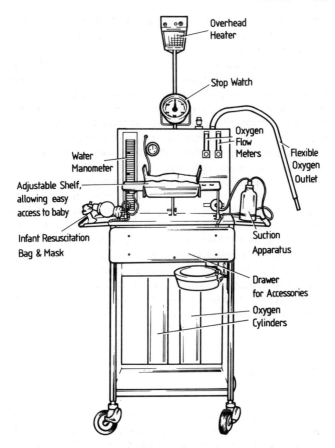

Fig. 11.4   The Resuscitaire—a typical infant resuscitation unit.

The third stage

There are various opinions on the subject of when the cord should be clamped and cut. If the baby requires active resuscitation then of course is must be clamped and cut immediately.

There are two methods of managing the third stage: active management and physiological management.

Active management This method was introduced relatively recently, in an attempt to reduce both the incidence and severity of postpartum haemorrhage. It was thought that shortening the third stage should tend to reduce blood loss for all women. However, women who wish to have as natural a labour as possible often request a physiological third stage, and so the whole question is under review. In order to manage the third stage actively, the midwife must:

Give an oxytocic drug, usually an ampoule of Syntometrine (containing oxytocin and ergometrine) by intramuscular injection.
Perform controlled cord traction (Fig. 11.5), which involves supporting the uterus through the lower abdominal wall with one hand, while grasping the cord with the other, and pulling steadily in a downwards direction.

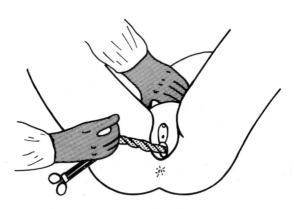

Fig. 11.5 Controlled cord traction.

Physiological management The midwife waits, without any kind of intervention, for the uterus to contract once more, though this may take an hour or more, and then asks the mother to bear down again; the placenta and membranes should then deliver spontaneously (Fig. 11.6).

The midwife gently swabs and inspects the perineum and the vaginal walls, checking to see if there are any lacerations requiring suturing. She then washes the vulval area, places a sterile pad over the vulva, and removes all wet or soiled linen, to make the mother comfortable. She checks the mother's blood pressure, temperature and pulse, and if all is well, gives the couple a cup of tea.

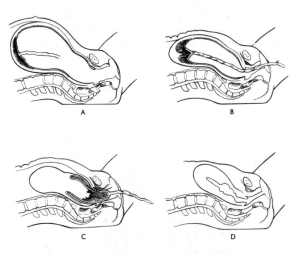

Fig. 11.6 The mechanism of placental separation. A, The placenta before the child is born; B, The placenta partially separated immediately after the birth of the child; C, the placenta completely separated; D, the placenta expelled and the uterus strongly contracted and retracted.

CARE IN THE IMMEDIATE POSTPARTUM PERIOD

While the new family have some time together, un-disturbed if possible, the midwife completes the case notes, which must include a birth notification form to the Registrar of Births and Deaths, and an entry in a register of cases.

Any perineal or vaginal repairs required should then be carried out, so that the time lapse is not too great. Ideally the midwife will perform the suturing, but whoever does so, it must be done with great care, in the interests of aligning the pelvic floor muscles ac-curately, and preventing subsequent problems, such as dyspareunia, stress incontinence, and later prolapse.

If the mother is fit and well, she may then get up and have a bath or shower, otherwise she will be helped to wash in bed. She is encouraged to pass urine; she will find this easier if she is able to get up. The amount passed is usually recorded, since it is im-portant to recognize any difficulties with micturition.

FURTHER CARE OF THE BABY

The main principle in care of the new baby is pre-vention of chilling. As already described, he is dried thoroughly at delivery, and if then covered with warm blankets and placed in skin-to-skin contact with his mother, he will usually remain warm, provided the room is warm and draught-free.

He will usually be alert and responsive during the first hour of life, and will usually feed well, so he may be put to the breast if the mother wishes.

The midwife will examine the baby systematically, checking to see that he appears normal. She notes his general appearance, and then examines him from head to toe. She will check his reflex responses (de-

scribed in Chapter 16—'The Normal Baby'). It is helpful to do all this in front of the parents, taking the
opportunity to point out to them just how aware their
baby is, and how much he is able to do.

The midwife weighs the baby and measures his
head circumference and length. She attaches identity
labels to the baby's wrist and ankle, checking the details with the mother against her own identity band.

Babies in the UK are usually given a dose of vitamin
K, either orally or intramuscularly, and this is discussed with the parents. It is given because the gut
flora necessary for its production are not present at
birth, but the liver requires vitamin K for the synthesis
of certain clotting factors.

If he has not already fed, the baby is offered a feed,
and if the parents do not wish to cuddle the baby
again, he is tucked down in a warm cot.

Before mother and baby are transferred to the postnatal ward together, the ward staff are given all the
relevant details.

FURTHER READING

FLINT, C. (1986) *Sensitive Midwifery*. London: Heinemann.

LLEWELLYN-JONES, D. (1982) *Fundamentals of Obstetrics and Gynaecology*,
Vol. I, 3rd edn, London: Faber & Faber.

MATERNITY SERVICES ADVISORY COMMITTEE (1984) *Maternity Care in
Action (Part II—Care in Labour)*. London: HMSO.

ODENT, M. (1984) *Birth Reborn*. London: Souvenir Press.

O'DRISCOLL, K. & MEAGHER, D. (1986) *Active Management of Labour*,
2nd edn. London: Baillière Tindall.

STANWAY, A. & STANWAY, P. (1984) *Choices in Childbirth*. London:
Pan Books.

SWEET, B. R. (1988) *Mayes' Midwifery—a Textbook for Midwives*, 11th
edn. London: Baillière Tindall.

12

ABNORMAL LABOUR

Part of the midwife's remit is to care for women in normal labour; she is expected to detect any abnormality and call for medical aid. The obstetrician then assumes responsibility for the woman's care, and he and the midwife work together.

Some definitions

Induction of labour This is the term used when labour is made to commence using artificial means.

Augmentation of labour This is the term used when labour, already in progress, is speeded up, or assisted, using artificial means.

INDUCTION OF LABOUR

This is usually described as medical or surgical.

'Medical' induction of labour This involves the use of hormones—either prostaglandin or oxytocin. It is common nowadays to give prostaglandin E2 as a pessary or gel. This aids 'ripening' of the cervix (the 'ripe' cervix is soft, often partially effaced, and ready to dilate) and when the cervix is favourable, will stimulate the commencement of effective uterine contractions.

Occasionally intravenous prostaglandin E2 or F2 may be used, but this is more common in early pregnancy, since it is more effective than oxytocin in termination of pregnancy. It often causes nausea and vomiting.

Intravenous oxytocin may be commended immediately after artificial rupture of the membranes, or after a period of, say, four hours. It is more commonly seen in augmentation than in induction of labour since prostaglandins came into wide use.

Administration of synthetic oxytocin (Syntocinon) is carefully controlled, and measured dosages are given with the help of an electronic drip counter or pump. The amount given is increased steadily, but not too rapidly. The fetal heart rate is monitored continuously, and the strength, duration and frequency of uterine contractions noted. Over-stimulation of the uterus will result in hypertonic contractions, which will be painful and distress the mother, as well as tending to cause fetal hypoxia because of reduced placental perfusion during uterine contractions.

The blood pressure is recorded every half hour. (Hourly recordings are sufficient in normal labour.) It is usual to run a 'main line' infusion of crystalloid solution as well as the oxytocin infusion, in order to keep the mother well hydrated and to keep the vein patent if the oxytocin infusion is discontinued temporarily because of hypertonic contractions.

'Surgical' induction of labour   This is performed by rupturing the membranes, usually the forewaters (that part of the amniotic sac felt in front of the presenting part).

Induction of labour is performed more selectively than was the case even a few years ago. The condition of the fetus may now be assessed and monitored much more accurately with ultrasound scanning widely available. Gestational age may also be assessed much more accurately, and it is always very important to know this, so that preterm delivery is avoided unless essential in the interests of either mother or baby. If preterm delivery is necessary, a knowledge of the gestational age helps the paediatrician to give the parents a realistic prognosis for the baby.

Indications

Postmaturity—if there are signs of placental deterioration.
Pregnancy-induced hypertension.
Placental insufficency.
Fetal abnormality.
Intrauterine death.
Medical problems in the mother—these include diabetes and renal disease.
Rhesus incompatibility—this is rare with modern preventive measures.

MALPRESENTATION

This was discussed in Chapter 10—'Problems in Later Pregnancy'.
Malpresentations are:

breech
face
brow
shoulder presentations

Any woman in labour with a breech or face presentation may have a vaginal delivery, but may need to have an emergency caesarean section at any time. A primigravida is likely to have a caesarean section immediately. A woman in labour with a brow or shoulder

presentation normally has a caesarean section as soon
as the presentation is diagnosed.

Nursing needs

These are as for normal labour, plus:

> Encouragement, reassurance and full explanations—
> these are needed throughout, even more than for
> the woman in normal labour. She should be pre-
> pared for the possibility of caesarean section.
> Sips of water or ice to suck; she may not eat.
> Regular antacid therapy (see page 174).
> Continuous fetal monitoring.
> Effective analgesia—epidural analgesia is often
> recommended but the mother should not be coerced.

An important stimulant to uterine contractions is
thought to be pressure from the presenting part on
the cervix. If the breech or face is presenting, this
stimulus is often less effective because the presenting
part fits less well, and so augmentation of labour with
an oxytocin infusion is commonly required.

MALPOSITION

This is defined and described in Chapter 10—'Problems
in Later Pregnancy'.

An occipito-posterior position of the head tends to
result in prolonged labour, and the woman is often
distressed by severe backache. This labour commonly
requires augmentation, and the woman will need
effective analgesia when possible, though even epidural analgesia will not always alleviate the backache
successfully. The mother with an occipito-posterior
position therefore requires much support and encour-

agement through what is often an exhausting, slow labour. Skill and ingenuity is needed to find different positions which may give a degree of relief, or temporary comfort.

There may be one of two outcomes:

1. The fetal head may rotate to an occipito-anterior position resulting in a normal delivery, or an uncomplicated, non-rotational forceps delivery.

2. The fetal head may remain in the occipito-posterior position, resulting in a 'face to pubes' or 'persistent occipito-posterior' delivery. This may be described as a spontaneous vaginal delivery, but is not a normal delivery. There will often be delay in the second stage, and forceps delivery is frequently necessary. The obstetrician examines the mother very carefully to define the position correctly, and to assess the likelihood of an uncomplicated forceps delivery. He then rotates the baby's head, either with forceps (see page 168), or manually, before delivering the baby. If there is any chance that the forceps delivery will be unsuccessful or difficult, the woman has an immediate caesarean section.

CEPHALOPELVIC DISPROPORTION

This was discussed briefly in Chapter 10—'Problems in Later Pregnancy'.

Definite cephalopelvic disproportion requires caesarean section, but if there is only a mild degree, with a good chance of successful vaginal delivery, the woman may have a 'trial of labour'. This involves giving the woman a predetermined time in established labour, using oxytocin if necessary. If progress, defined by cervical dilatation and descent of the fetal head, is good, and vaginal delivery seems likely, she will be allowed to continue. If there is any doubt about the outcome, caesarean section is performed.

PREGNANCY-INDUCED HYPERTENSION

The woman with mild pregnancy-induced hypertension needs careful monitoring of her blood pressure during labour, but otherwise needs no special care or treatment. If her blood pressure rises significantly, or the cardiotocograph becomes abnormal, the obstetrician must be informed immediately.

The woman with moderate to severe pregnancy-induced hypertension requires more special care. She must have a midwife with her constantly, and must be watched closely for signs of fulminating pre-eclampsia (see Chapter 10, 'Problems in Later Pregnancy'). Labour is often induced, particularly as the placenta may show signs of deterioration before term, and fetal growth may slow down. An intravenous infusion is commenced, so that drug therapy may be given as necessary.

Observations

Observations are as in normal labour plus:

Continual fetal monitoring.
Blood pressure is recorded every 15 to 30 minutes.
Central venous pressure (CVP) recordings if a CVP line has been inserted.
Fluid balance.
Urinalysis, with quantitative estimation of albuminuria, using Esbach's test.
Inspection and estimation of oedema.
Record level of consciousness if the patient is under heavy sedation.

Medication

Drugs given may include the following.

Anti-hypertensives Hydralazine or labetalol are currently in use.

Sedatives These are given if an eclamptic fit occurs or seems imminent because the woman is restless and hyperreflexic. Chlormethiazole is an anti-convulsant as well as a sedative. Diazepam may be used, but is preferred by some after delivery, because of its effect on the fetus. 'Lytic cocktail' is a traditional treatment, but may still be seen occasionally; it contains chlorpromazine, promethazine and pethidine. It will have a depressant effect on the fetus, and again, is best used after delivery.

Diuretics These may be of some benefit. One of the complications of pregnancy-induced hypertension is poor renal function.

Antibiotics These may be prescribed to prevent hypostatic pneumonia.

Nursing needs

All care is as for a woman in labour, as described in Chapter 10—'Normal labour', plus:

  Constant surveillance in a calm, peaceful atmosphere, with minimal disturbance and handling.
  Pressure area care, with regular turning.
  Regular mouth care.
  Eye care, keeping the lids shut, and instilling hypromellose drops if necessary.
  Maintain a clear airway.

Give all drugs as prescribed.
Inform medical staff of all developments.
Keep the woman's partner fully involved and in-formed; he will need much reassurance.

An eclamptic fit closely resembles an epileptic fit.

Care during a fit

Maintain a clear airway, using suction equipment if necessary, and turning the patient into the 're-covery' position.
Give oxygen if necessary.
Call medical aid.
Protect the woman from injury.
Note the duration of the fit, and the signs preceding it.

When an eclamptic fit has occurred, the woman must be delivered as soon as possible. (The symptoms may be controlled to some extent, but the only cure for the condition itself is delivery of the baby.) There is a risk of placental abruption following a fit, so the fetal heart must be monitored continually.
Complications for the mother include:

Impaired renal function, or renal failure.
Disseminated intravascular coagulation (DIC).
Risk of cerebrovascular accident if the blood pressure remains high and uncontrolled.

COMPLICATIONS DURING NORMAL LABOUR

Complications may arise at any time in a previously normal labour.

Fetal distress

Cardiotocography and its interpretation is discussed in Chapter 11—'Normal Labour'. Fetal distress is suspected on abnormal cardiotocography and meconium-stained liquor, and confirmed by fetal blood sampling.

Abnormal cardiotocography   Type II dips, or late decelerations, are dips in the fetal heart tracing which occur late in relation to the peak of the contraction. The later they occur, and the longer their duration, the more ominous they are. If associated with a 'flat' trace, that is, one showing little beat to beat variability, they are even more ominous.

Meconium staining of the liquor   The hypoxic fetus will pass meconium *in utero*. The only time meconium staining may be regarded as normal is in breech presentation, when pressure on the presenting part may cause meconium to be squeezed out. This is why it is important to observe the colour of the liquor throughout labour. If meconium is present, the midwife must decide whether it is stale or fresh, and whether there is just a trace, or whether the liquor is heavily stained.

Fetal blood sampling   In this procedure a drop of capillary blood is taken from the fetus's scalp, using a special instrument called an amnioscope which has a light source. The doctor can then visualize the presenting part through the os. The pH of the blood sample is measured, giving an indication of the degree of acidosis if the fetus is becoming hypoxic.

The whole situation is assessed by these three parameters, taking into account the woman's parity and how imminent delivery is. If fetal distress is severe, and the cervix is not fully dilated, immediate caesarean section is performed. If the cervix is fully dilated, the baby may be delivered by forceps.

Failure to progress

This term may be used to describe events in the first or second stage of labour, but the two problems are somewhat different.

Failure to progress in the first stage of labour   This is usually due to incoordinate, or disordered uterine action, when contractions may be strong, frequent and very painful, but are ineffective because there is little or no cervical dilatation. As already discussed, delay may be due to malpresentation or malposition.

Failure to progress in the second stage of labour   If the cervix is fully dilated, then the uterine contractions have been co-ordinated and effective. Sometimes there may be a degree of uterine inertia in the second stage, and augmentation with oxytocin may be helpful. The second stage of labour is often prolonged by an occipito-posterior position of the head. The duration of the second stage itself is less significant than the length of time the woman has been actively pushing. If the active phase lasts more than about an hour without good progress, the woman will become exhausted, and the fetus is likely to become hypoxic. The baby is normally delivered by forceps in this case.

INSTRUMENTAL DELIVERY

Forceps delivery

Forceps delivery may be described as rotational or non-rotational. If the fetal head is in any position other than occipito-anterior, it is best rotated gently before delivery.

Obstetric forceps vary in design depending on their intended use, but the general principles are the same.

All are designed to grasp the baby's head without causing trauma, if correctly applied.

Forceps designed for non-rotational delivery include: Wrigley's, Neville-Barnes' and Anderson's.

Forceps designed for rotation of the fetal head are the Kielland's (or Kjelland's) forceps.

Before the obstetrician performs a forceps delivery, he ensures that:

The cervix is fully dilated.
The woman has adequate analgesia.
Her bladder is empty.
He is sure of the position of the baby's head.
He is likely to be able to deliver the baby without pulling hard.
Everything he requires is at hand.
The paediatrician is present if required.

The couple must have had as full an explanation as they require. When all equipment and personnel are ready, the woman is placed in the lithotomy position. The vulval area is cleaned and draped, the forceps blades are gently inserted, one at a time, on either side of the fetal head. The midwife who has been caring for the woman gives her her undivided attention and support, and encourages her to bear down with the contractions as soon as the doctor is ready. He then exerts steady, downwards traction on the forceps until the head crowns, and the rest of the delivery follows the normal pattern.

Only on very rare occasions is a forceps delivery performed without an episiotomy. The perineum is usually repaired while the woman is in the lithotomy position, with the analgesia given for delivery still effective.

Caesarean section

Caesarean section is described as 'lower segment' or classical. The lower segment of the uterus forms during the last weeks of pregnancy, and has its muscle fibres arranged rather differently to those in the upper segment. If a uterine incision is made in the lower segment it bleeds less, heals better and is less prone to rupture in a subsequent pregnancy. A classical caesarean section is performed in the woman whose pregnancy has only reached about 32 weeks or less, simply because there is no lower segment, or in cases of anterior placenta praevia, where there is a real risk of cutting through the placenta.

The student may find it confusing that there are two types of incision, a Pfannenstiel or 'bikini line', and a midline. A lower segment caesarean section may be performed through either type of incision, whereas a classical caesarean section always necessitates a mid-line approach. It is wrong, therefore, to assume that because the scar is a midline one, this was a classical caesarean section.

Caesarean section may be performed under general anaesthesia or epidural or spinal anaesthesia. Very occasionally it may be performed under local anaesthesia, and of course this technique has its uses in the remote situation, without the help of an anaesthetist.

Despite all the advances of recent years, obstetric anaesthesia still has its particular hazards, and many anaesthetists would prefer women to have epidural anaesthesia. However, it is not appropriate to persuade women, and they must be counselled rather than coerced. Regional anaesthesia (epidural or spinal) has the advantage that the woman can see and cuddle her baby as soon as he is born, and in many centres the baby's father can also be present. Women recovering from general anaesthesia have difficulty recalling events, and distinguishing dream from reality. Some have said that they had delay or difficulty forming an attachment with the baby because of this.

Breech delivery

Breech delivery is described as follows.

Assisted breech delivery The baby's body is born spontaneously, and then the head is delivered in a carefully controlled manner, usually with forceps, but sometimes using one of two special techniques,

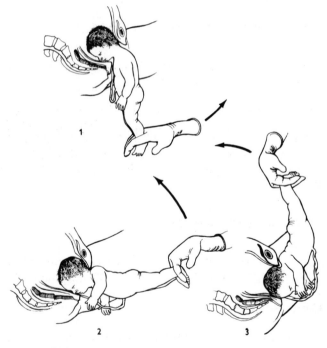

Fig. 12.1 The Burns–Marshall manoeuvre.

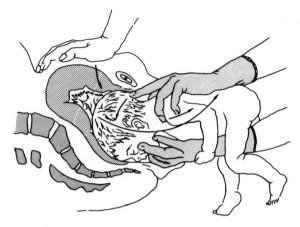

Fig. 12.2   The Mauriceau–Smellie–Veit manoeuvre.

the Burns–Marshall or Mauriceau–Smellie–Veit ma-
noeuvres (Figs. 12.1 and 12.2).

Breech extraction   This term is used to describe breech
delivery under general anaesthetic, where the body is
not born spontaneously. It is rarely seen nowadays in
the UK. If delivery is likely to be at all difficult, caesarean section is performed, as it is less hazardous for
the baby.

OBSTETRIC EMERGENCIES

There are certain situations in obstetrics which require
immediate recognition and prompt and urgent action.

Cord prolapse

If the presenting part is high in the pelvic brim and the
membranes rupture, the umbilical cord may be swept

down with the gush of liquor. If the presenting part then descends into the pelvis the resulting cord compression will lead to fetal hypoxia. The woman's bed is tilted head down, or she may be positioned in the knee–chest position. The midwife will scrub and put on sterile gloves, and hold the presenting part off the cord. Caesarean section is performed as quickly as possible. In cord presentation the cord is felt lying in front of the presenting part through intact membranes on vaginal examination. Obviously if the membranes rupture, this will become a cord prolapse. The fetal heart must be monitored to detect any fetal distress resulting from cord compression.

Shoulder dystocia

With a large or abnormal baby the shoulders may become impacted beneath the mother's symphysis pubis. Medical help is needed urgently, but meantime, placing the woman in the lithotomy position often allows delivery of the shoulders. The baby's clavicles may be fractured in the attempt.

Severe haemorrhage

Haemorrhage may occur during pregnancy (see chapters 9 and 10), during labour or following delivery (see page 175).

PERINEAL DAMAGE

Perineal damage is not abnormal unless it is severe.
    A perineal tear is described as follows.

First degree   The skin only is involved.

Second degree   The skin and muscle layers are involved.

Third degree   The tear extends to the anal sphincter. This type of tear must be repaired with great care; it is carried out under general or regional anaesthesia. The woman will require analgesia in the postnatal period, and it is usual to give a stool softener, such as Mil-Par.

OBSTETRIC ANAESTHESIA

This is discussed in this chapter, as general anaesthesia is often required to deal with situations in abnormal labour. Obstetric anaesthesia is potentially hazardous, and requires an experienced anaesthetist with specialist knowledge. The problems encountered arise largely from the following factors:

The effects of progesterone on plain muscle.
The physical pressure on the diaphragm and thoracic cavity from the pregnant uterus.
The unique situation of having two patients—mother and baby.

Progesterone effects on plain muscle   The most important of these is the effect on the musculature of the stomach. Gastric motility is markedly reduced in labour, so that the stomach remains full, even though the woman may not have eaten for some hours. These stomach contents will become very acid because they are not being digested and moved on. Progesterone also renders the sphincters relatively incompetent.

Problems in obstetric anaesthesia

Mendelson's syndrome   If the stomach is full of acid contents, with a lax sphincter, and pressure from the gravid uterus in the recumbent position, silent regurgitation of stomach contents can easily occur. If this acid material is inhaled it leads to a chemical pneumonitis; the woman becomes critically ill, and may die. Antacids are given to women in labour in order to raise the pH of the stomach contents, so that damage to the lungs is likely to be less severe if inhalation should occur.

Failed intubation   Because of the very real risk of 'silent aspiration', leading to Mendelson's syndrome, every pregnant woman having a general anaesthetic in the second or third trimester of pregnancy, or in the first 48 hours following delivery, should have 'crash induction' anaesthesia, with cricoid pressure and endotracheal intubation. Because the pregnant woman at term usually has a degree of generalized oedema the anaesthetist may have difficulty visualizing the trachea and vocal cords. The problem may be compounded by large breasts or general obesity making the application of cricoid pressure difficult. (Cricoid pressure is a technique which uses pressure on the cricoid cartilage, a complete ring of tracheal cartilage, to occlude the oesophagus, and so prevent gastric reflux.)

Aortocaval occlusion   This is a risk at any time during the last weeks of pregnancy. If the woman lies recumbent, the weight of the gravid uterus pressing on the vena cava may reduce venous return, thus reducing cardiac output, thus reducing placental blood flow. It is now recognized that there may be an adverse effect on the fetus before there are signs or symptoms of a fall in maternal blood pressure. An episode of fetal hypoxia is not desirable before either epidural or general anaesthesia, so this is something of which anaesthetists are particularly aware.

Maternal awareness Because of the possibility of producing respiratory depression and sleepiness in the newborn baby, the anaesthetist gives the mother a fairly light anaesthetic prior to delivery of the baby. She will be paralysed, because she has an endotracheal tube in position, and a muscle relaxant is given in order to intubate, and so she may occasionally be aware of what is going on around her but be unable to move, or otherwise indicate her predicament. The anaesthetist has a responsibility to try to prevent this nightmarish situation occurring, and anaesthetic techniques for caesarean section have been evolved with this in mind.

THE THIRD STAGE

There are two main problems which may arise in the third stage of labour: postpartum haemorrhage and retained placenta.

Postpartum haemorrhage

This is defined as excessive bleeding from the genital tract following delivery of the baby. It is described as primary or secondary.

Primary postpartum haemorrhage occurs in the first 24 hours following delivery; after this time it is known as secondary.

Secondary postpartum haemorrhage may occur up to six weeks after delivery. It is usually associated with uterine infection, which is turn is usually associated with retained products of conception. Even a tiny fragment of placental tissue or membrane can lead to this complication, and so it is very important to ascertain whether or not the placenta and membranes are complete following delivery.

Postpartum haemorrhage may occur suddenly and dramatically; a woman may lose an alarming amount of blood in a very short time. The midwife must respond promptly and appropriately, since haemorrhage may be fatal.

Immediate first aid depends on whether or not the uterus is relaxed. The midwife will send an urgent message, summoning medical aid; she will attempt to 'rub up' a uterine contraction, and may also give a second dose of Syntometrine, the oxytocic preparation used in active management of the third stage (see page 154). If the uterus is already well contracted, or the treatment described has no effect, it is important to ascertain exactly where the bleeding originates. Sometimes a vaginal or cervical tear, previously missed, may be bleeding profusely. In this case, immediate suturing is required. Blood loss must be estimated as accurately as possible, and fluid loss replaced.

Severe blood loss may lead to disseminated intravascular coagulation (DIC) or renal failure.

Any retained products of conception must be evacuated from the uterus, under regional or general anaesthesia.

Retained placenta

Sometimes the midwife may not be able to deliver the placenta. This may be because:

A full bladder may impede separation and delivery of the placenta.
The placenta is trapped behind a closed cervix if the cervix clamps down quickly.

The cord may snap during controlled cord traction. Occasionally the placenta is truly adherent, and does not separate from the uterine wall. Only very rarely indeed is placenta accreta seen; in this complication the placenta has embedded deeply into the uterine wall, and hysterectomy is necessary.

The obstetrician is informed if the placenta is not delivered within 20–30 minutes in active management of the third stage, and within 60–75 minutes in physiological management. If there is no undue blood loss, he may wait a further time before preparing to remove the placenta manually, under regional or general anaesthesia. This procedure becomes an urgent matter if the woman starts to bleed.

FURTHER READING

BEVIS, R. (1984) *Anaesthesia in Midwifery*. London: Baillière Tindall.

DONALD, I. (1979) *Practical Obstetric Problems*. London: Lloyd-Luke Medical Books.

LLEWELLYN-JONES, D. (1986) *Fundamentals of Obstetrics and Gynaecology*, Vol. I, 3rd edn. London: Faber & Faber.

SWEET, B. R. (1986) *Mayes' Midwifery—a Textbook for Midwives*, 10th edn. London: Baillière Tindall.

13

PAIN RELIEF IN LABOUR

SOME DEFINITIONS

Analgesia   This is absence of pain.

Anaesthesia   This is absence of sensation.

It is important to appreciate the difference between these two terms, and to use them correctly.

PHYSIOLOGY OF PAIN

Perception of pain is influenced by such factors as anxiety and fear, expectation, cultural behaviour and the environment. Painful sensations may be clearly defined, so that the sufferer can describe the sensation and the exact location. This tends to occur in acute pain, often from trauma. Such pain sensations are transmitted along myelinated nerve fibres, known as A fibres.

Chronic pain sensations are transmitted along un-myelinated C fibres; such impulses are transmitted more slowly and the sensation is often less well defined.

Pain from the abdominal organs is not well defined, and is sometimes called visceral pain. Pain may be appreciated at some point other than that which is diseased or damaged; this is 'referred pain'.

The transmission of the pain stimulus, and its inter-pretation in the sensory cortex is described as the 'pain pathway'. The pain pathway consists of the sensory nerve receiving the painful stimulus; this travels to the posterior or dorsal root ganglion of the spinal cord, and thence to the posterior horn. This is described as the 'first neurone'. The sensation then ascends through the spinal cord, to the medulla, pons varolii and mid-brain to the thalamus—the 'second neurone'. Finally it traverses the 'third neurone', to reach the cerebral cortex, where it is interpreted, and the subject responds vocally or by taking evasive action.

PAIN IN LABOUR

The unique, intense and protracted pain of labour arises from the following causes.

Uterine contractions   These cause an ischaemic type of pain which is not clearly localized, and is usually described by the woman as 'like a bad period pain'. It may also be referred to the groins and the top of the thighs. Women often expect to feel it over the uterine fundus, but the sensation is usually over the lower abdomen. They frequently complain of backache, or back pain.

Cervical dilatation   This also contributes to the lower abdominal and back pain. The spinal nerves involved in both the pain arising from uterine contractions and cervical dilatation are T11 and T12, and in the later stages of labour, T10 and L1 are also involved.

Stretching of the vagina and its surrounding structures, and finally the perineum   This is usually very painful, although it may be described as an unpleasant burning, stretching sensation with intense rectal pressure. At this stage all the lumbar and sacral nerves are involved.

INTERVENTION

Pain may be treated by arresting or interrupting transmission of the pain stimulus at various points.

At the receptor site   This is effected by the use of local anaesthetic solution, for example prior to performing an episiotomy or suturing.

At the point where the first and second neurones meet This is achieved by the use of regional anaesthesia; this may be epidural or spinal block.

At a cerebral level   Methods used include systemic analgesics, such as the opiates, inhalational analgesia, and general anaesthesia.

There are also physiological mechanisms for coping with pain. The body is able to produce its own opiates in response to pain. These are called endogenous opiates, and are subdivided into endorphins and enkephalins.

Since the subject's reaction to pain is conditioned to some extent by cultural and social norms and expectations, and by her mental and emotional state, there is a definite psychological component in pain relief.

PSYCHOLOGICAL PREPARATION FOR LABOUR

Women need to be prepared for the almost inevitable pain of labour since only a very small minority enjoy a painless experience without analgesia.

The objective is not to frighten women, but to prepare them realistically, to reassure them that they will be able to cope, and that there are varied means of relief available to them. Total freedom from pain cannot be promised, since this is not realistic, but it should be possible to promise that the woman will not be left alone during her labour. It has been shown that the presence of a supportive companion significantly reduces the need for pain relief. Part of the reasoning behind relaxation classes is to give the woman a means of helping herself and making a positive contribution to coping with her labour.

Since fear of the unknown will play a large part in the woman's apprehension, much may be done by giving information, and allowing her to become familiar with the place which will be her environment during labour. The ideal is that she should also meet the midwife who will care for her, and that the same midwife should be with her throughout her labour. Continuity of care in the antenatal period is also helpful, since the woman is more likely to become relaxed and feel able to ask questions.

It is important that staff should be friendly and approachable, and that the environment should be pleasant and comfortable. Women and their partners should feel that they have an important contribution to make in deciding on and carrying out the details of their care, so that they do not feel that someone in authority has taken them over, and they have lost control.

Some of these factors may seem trivial, but they combine to make the difference between a good and a bad experience for the couple.

INHALATIONAL ANALGESIA

There are certain substances which, given in large doses, afford anaesthesia, and in small doses, analgesia.

The one substance in common use in the UK is Entonox, which is a mixture of equal parts of nitrous oxide and oxygen. It is the nitrous oxide which has the anaesthetic/analgesic properties, and its action is altered by increasing the ratio of nitrous oxide to oxygen. Midwives are trained in the administration of Entonox, and may then use it without medical supervision for women in labour, within certain rules laid down by their national and local governing bodies. Until a few years ago there were other substances which could be administered by the midwife, without medical supervision. These were trichloroethylene (Trilene) and methoxyflurane (Penthrane), which are still useful in the more remote situation.

Inhalational analgesia is given on a self-administration basis, so that if the woman has slightly too much, she will drop the mask, and will then quickly recover, since nitrous oxide is excreted in a very short time. It is important that the woman's partner, and indeed, the student nurse, should understand this principle, and encourage the woman to take the Entonox herself. In order to prevent overdose, the equipment is designed in such a way that the gas does not flow, but must be extracted by the woman's inspiratory effort.

The woman should be instructed carefully in the use of the Entonox, or she may not obtain real benefit from it. She should start to inhale from the mask as soon as she feels the contraction starting, and continue to take steady, deep breaths until the peak of the contraction has passed. There is a danger of hyperventilation, and women often blame the Entonox itself for the tingling face and fingers, and the dizziness.

Some women feel claustrophobic using a mask, and a special mouth-piece is available as an alternative.

THE OPIATES

Systemic analgesia may be used, giving an intramuscular injection of a morphine derivative. The most commonly used is pethidine, which has been in general use for many years, and despite much research to find a substitute, is still probably the most useful. The problem with giving opiates to the mother is that they tend to produce respiratory depression in the neonate. They are therefore used with great care. An opiate is not normally given within three to four hours of the anticipated time of delivery, and the total dose given during labour does not normally exceed a locally agreed amount (though this will vary).

The experienced midwife will not be alarmed if the woman progresses quickly in labour after receiving pethidine; the analgesia and consequent relaxation often has this effect. Even if the baby is sleepy at delivery, he is usually resuscitated easily, unless there is also some other cause. Neonatal naloxone may be given to reverse the respiratory depression if necessary. The after-effects of opiates which concern paediatricians, and sometimes parents, are much more subtle, but possibly more long-lived.

Some doctors like to use diamorphine for analgesia in labour, since it gives the woman a pleasant feeling of euphoria and detachment, but others fear the possibility of addiction.

The action of an opiate is potentiated by also giving promazine or promethazine. Some feel that promazine and promethazine reduce the incidence of nausea and vomiting, but it is probably better to give an antiemetic if this effect is required. Other opiate-like drugs which may be used are pentazocine (Fortral), which was never widely used, and meptazinol.

Midwives may give pain relief to women in labour, according to 'standing orders' laid down by the obstetricians in the Maternity Unit, and these standing orders usually include an opiate, with clearly defined parameters as to how much may be given. If a woman requires more than this permitted dose, the obstetrician must be consulted.

REGIONAL ANALGESIA

Epidural block

Surrounding the outer covering of the spinal cord, the dura mater, is the epidural space. The spinal nerves pass through this space, and it is possible to introduce local anaesthetic solution, which will bathe these nerves, and so produce selective anaesthesia (Fig. 13.1).

Epidural block for labour is performed at the intervertebral space between L1 and L2, L2 and L3, or L3 and L4 in order to produce analgesia at the right level.

Some women are very frightened of the idea of epidural anaesthesia, and are afraid that they will remain paralysed. This is a very minimal risk, but women must be carefully informed of what is involved in an epidural block, and should be given an opportunity to ask questions. They should not be persuaded against their will.

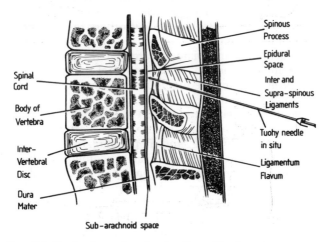

Fig. 13.1 The lumbar spine showing the epidural space.

An intravenous infusion is always commenced, and about 500 ml of fluid such as Hartmann's solution is infused before the epidural block is instituted. This is because there will be a degree of sympathetic blockade, as well as sensory and motor block; this often results in a fall in blood pressure, and the 'pre-load' has a buffering effect. It is for this reason that the blood pressure is checked frequently.

The anaesthetist will want the woman to lie on her left side, with her legs drawn up, or sitting upright on the bed, with her legs over the side, resting on a stool (Fig. 13.2).

The procedure is performed under strict aseptic technique.

It is essential for the anaesthetist to identify the

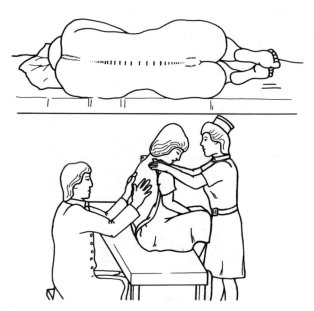

Fig. 13.2 Positioning of the patient prior to epidural analgesia.

epidural space correctly. He gives a 'test dose' of local anaesthetic solution first, and when he is satisfied that there are no adverse effects, he will give the remainder of the first dose. He will usually insert an epidural catheter, a very fine catheter, so that further doses of local anaesthetic solution may be given throughout the labour, to maintain adequate analgesia. The epidural catheter is securely strapped in position, with its length brought up the woman's back, and over her shoulder. An antibacterial filter is attached to the end of the catheter.

The anaesthetist gives the first dose of local anaesthetic solution, but then, depending on local policy, he may delegate further 'topping up' of the epidural to the midwife, if she is suitably trained and experienced. She is responsible for informing him if there is any kind of problem or complication.

For some women this is the ideal form of pain relief. Others may dislike the heaviness, tingling or immobility of the legs. The local anaesthetic solution most commonly used is bupivacaine (Marcain). This is supplied in solutions of 0.25% and 0.5%, but may be modified to 0.125% or 0.375% as required by dilution with sterile normal saline. Lignocaine may also be used in the epidural space. It is effective more quickly, but its effect is more short-lived, and so it is not considered suitable for prolonged use throughout labour, since a larger total dose will need to be given.

Nursing needs

Bladder care The woman will probably lose the sensation of a full bladder, and a bedpan should be offered every two hours.

The legs If the legs are numb and immobile, care must be taken to see that they do not suffer damage from pressure, or from resting in an unnatural position.

Position and comfort   The woman will need help to move around on the bed.

Analgesia   An adequate level of analgesia must be maintained, and the midwife 'tops up' the epidural on her own responsibility, or calls the anaesthetist to do so as appropriate.

Careful observation   The woman may have no sensation of wanting to bear down when she reaches the second stage of labour, and so the midwife watches closely for clinical signs of full dilatation of the cervix.

Blood pressure   This is recorded every half hour, and more frequently following further doses of local anaesthetic solution.

The intravenous infusion   This is an important adjunct to the epidural block, and it must be maintained with care.

The epidural catheter   This must be protected from becoming misplaced. The woman will be hot, and will perspire during labour, so that the strapping over the catheter may sometimes become loose.

Psychological   Once the woman is free from pain, she may sometimes begin to feel guilty that she has 'opted out' of the full experience of labour, particularly if she had intended not to have an epidural block.

Epidural block for caesarean section

Caesarean section may be performed under epidural anaesthesia. The block needed is much more profound and extensive, so the risk of hypotension is much greater, and the motor block in the legs is usually complete. The anaesthesia must reach nipple level, in order to block pain during the operation, but of course must not extend further, or the woman will begin to have difficulty in breathing. Women are often very 'shivery' at some stage during preparation for the caesarean section, and sometimes afterwards. The reason for this is unclear.

For most women who want this form of anaesthesia it is very satisfactory, as they can see and cuddle the baby immediately he is delivered, and may often have their partner with them.

Opiates given via the epidural route give very effective post-operative pain relief, and in some centres this will be available to women following caesarean section. The advantage is that there is no motor block, so that the woman may move her legs freely, thus minimizing the risk of deep vein thrombosis. Because she is pain-free and not sleepy, she will also be able to mobilize more quickly.

A combination of local anaesthetic solution and an opiate, such as fentanyl, has proved very effective, with fewer side effects. This combination is also used during labour.

If the caesarean section is urgent, for example because of severe fetal distress, there may not be time to perform epidural anaesthesia.

Complications of epidural anaesthesia

'Dural tap' If the anaesthetist inadvertently punctures the dura mater and therefore, almost inevitably, the arachnoid mater, so that cerebrospinal fluid (CSF) leaks out of the subarachnoid space, the woman is likely to suffer a headache, which is usually severe. The epidural catheter is resited, and the anaesthetist will often run an infusion of normal saline into the epidural space following delivery, in an attempt to maintain pressure within the space, and so minimize CSF leakage. He will not want the woman to bear down, and so an elective forceps delivery will be performed. He may also want the woman kept flat.

Total spinal   If a dural tap is undetected, and local anaesthetic solution for an epidural block is introduced into the subarachnoid space, the woman will suffer immediate, profound collapse, with severe hypotension, and sometimes cardiac arrest. She requires immediate, skilled resuscitation if she is to survive unscathed. This should be a very rare occurrence, but the possibility emphasizes the need for vigilant, experienced care.

'Bloody tap'   If the anaesthetist inadvertently punctures a blood vessel, he will perform the epidural block via another intervertebral space, to reduce the risk of introducing the local anaesthetic solution into the circulation.

Back pain following delivery   There may be a degree of local bruising and trauma where the epidural was sited, particularly if the anaesthetist had difficulty introducing the epidural (Tuohy) needle.

Difficulty with micturition   This may occur following any delivery, but is sometimes attributed to the loss of sensation following an epidural.

Headache   Some claim that this is a complication of epidural analgesia, but there is no well-founded reason for this, apart from dural tap, described above.

Spinal anaesthesia

It is important to distinguish spinal from epidural anaesthesia. In spinal or subarachnoid anaesthesia,

local anaesthetic solution is introduced into the subarachnoid space, in other words, into the CSF. Very
small amounts of local anaesthetic solution are required,
and a much finer needle is used, to minimize leakage
of CSF. Spinal anaesthesia gives rapid, effective anaesthesia, and so is useful for procedures such as
manual removal of a retained placenta, repair of a third
degree tear, or forceps delivery.

Some anaesthetists have evolved a technique for
caesarean section which combines spinal and epidural
anaesthesia. Immediate anaesthesia is given by the
'spinal', and anaesthesia is maintained by the epidural
block.

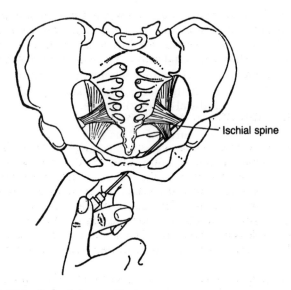

Fig. 13.3   Pudendal nerve block.

LOCAL ANAESTHESIA

Pudendal block In order to give adequate analgesia for a forceps delivery, some obstetricians will perform pudendal block (Fig. 13.3). The pudendal nerve lies adjacent to the sacro-spinous ligament. A long, guarded needle, called an Oxford needle, is used, and the usual approach is transvaginal, though it may also be performed transperineally. An effective pudendal block gives good perineal and vaginal anaesthesia, but this is often difficult to achieve, except in very experienced hands.

Paracervical block This is a more extensive block, where the paracervical plexus is anaesthetized. There are potential risks, and so it has never been widely used in the UK.

Perineal infiltration This is performed prior to making an episiotomy or suturing the perineum. Midwives in the UK are permitted to use this method of local anaesthesia. The drug most commonly used is lignocaine, 0.5% or 1%.

OTHER METHODS OF PAIN RELIEF

Transcutaneous nerve stimulation (TCNS or TENS) This is thought to utilize the 'gate control' mechanism. Electrodes are attached to the mother's back, and using a small battery-powered device, the woman is able to give herself a small, electrical impulse. She increases the intensity as much as is necessary, or until she finds it an unpleasant sensation. For some women it works well, and appears to be safe, and free from side effects.

Psychoprophylaxis This and other methods that have been developed along similar lines utilize the psychological approach, which theorizes that ignorance leads to fear, resulting in tension, in turn resulting in intensified pain. By giving information, allaying anxiety and teaching the principles of relaxation, the woman is enabled to feel more in control of the situation. There is also an element of distraction in these techniques.

Hypnosis   This may be suitable for some women. It is rarely available outside private practice.

Acupuncture   The main difficulty with this method of pain relief is likely to be finding a practitioner who is willing to be available whenever the woman goes into labour.

Homeopathy   Homeopaths offer remedies and treatments to help the woman before and during labour.

FURTHER READING

BEVIS, R. (1984) *Anaesthesia in Midwifery*. London, Baillière Tindall.
MOIR, D. (1980) *Obstetric Anaesthesia and Analgesia*, 2nd edn. London, Baillière Tindall.

14

POSTNATAL CARE

The postnatal period, or puerperium, may be defined as the time during which the new mother returns to 'normal', or to a state similar to her pre-pregnancy state, physically and emotionally. It is impossible to be categorical about this, since it may be argued that a woman is never the same once she has had a baby. The immediate postnatal period can reasonably be defined as the first 10 to 14 days following delivery, and the puerperium as a whole, the six weeks following delivery. It is important to appreciate that in some societies, the concept of 'lying in' or 'confinement' still applies, and that our Western ideas of being up and about so quickly seem literally very foreign, and quite improper.

Postnatal care is the most neglected aspect of obstetrics, yet it is an extremely significant period in every mother's life, particularly if she has just had her first baby.

Women are tending to be sent home earlier, to the care of the domiciliary midwife, often without a great deal of family support. Fewer women now have already had experience with a small baby, as they had in the prewar days of larger families. Little wonder, then, that the postnatal period is a time of great stress and uncertainty for many women.

For the professional woman, motherhood may be a devastating experience; this small person refuses to behave as the books suggest he should, and he will not be organized into a routine as her work and her colleagues would, when she was pursuing her career.

Spending her life at home, immersed in baby-care and domesticity, may become less attractive with the passage of time. For many women, motherhood is then not the lovely, romantic experience it appeared from a distance, but is remarkably exhausting and time-consuming.

The skill in postnatal care lies in knowing how much to do for each new mother, so as to give adequate support, without making the woman feel incompetent, or indeed, preventing her learning the new skills she must acquire.

MOTHER/BABY ATTACHMENT

The term 'bonding', popular until recently, has been replaced by the word 'attachment'.

Most women expect to feel an overwhelming rush of maternal feeling as soon as their new baby is placed in their arms. Many do not, and feel worried and guilty, but this is hardly surprising, after a lengthy, exhausting physical and emotional experience.

Mother/baby attachment is much more likely to grow and develop as time passes. Immediate attachment is like 'love at first sight'—it does happen, but not to most people. Having said this, the new baby is designed to look appealing. Adult humans are attracted to miniature versions of any animal, and the new baby's physical features and his dependence are attractive, as well as his cry being very difficult to ignore!

Prenatal factors have a part to play in this whole question, and the mother who has a supportive relationship with her partner, with no financial or social pressures, whose pregnancy was wanted and planned, is more likely to form a satisfying relationship with her baby.

Temperament also has a part to play, and the placid

woman is likely to settle into an enjoyable motherhood quickly.

Stress and tiredness are two factors which will tend to delay the formation of a satisfying mother/baby relationship. Those involved in postnatal care will therefore do well to try to prevent both from arising. 'Rooming-in' is the term used when the mother has her baby beside her, rather than in the nursery. It was a policy which came into vogue rather rapidly, as a result of 'bonding' theories. The woman who did not wish to have her baby with her day and night then tended to be viewed with some suspicion, as one who was not becoming properly attached! One pitfall with this system is that only the minority of women have a single room; indeed, many would feel shut away and isolated if they were given one. Many modern postnatal wards have four or six beds in each section or room, and so mothers' sleep is disturbed by other women's babies as well as their own.

Rooming in, then, is a policy which must be implemented with flexibility. Planned care should allow women to choose whether or not their babies remain with them day and night, and ward staff should be prepared to relieve the exhausted mother who needs a period of undisturbed sleep. Like many other hospital wards, the postnatal ward tends to be unnecessarily, and sometimes unavoidably, noisy at night, and perhaps women would be well advised to make use of ear-plugs with the proviso that the staff would wake her if she slept through her own baby's crying.

While mother/baby attachment is not attained overnight, the postnatal period is an important time for detecting a real lack of attachment. The mother who does not become attached to her baby in a way which is satisfying to both (not necessarily to the professionals!), and who does not display maternal behaviour, is more likely to abuse her child subsequently. The woman who behaves in an uncharacteristic fashion (for her) may be developing postnatal depression or puerperal psychosis.

ESTABLISHMENT OF FEEDING

This is an important aspect of postnatal care, which is discussed in more detail in Chapter 17—'Infant Feeding'.

PRACTICAL ASPECTS OF MOTHERHOOD

Although it will take most women some time before they handle a small baby confidently, the mother must have acquired certain skills and knowledge before she returns home. She needs to be able to mix an artificial feed and should know how to sterilize the feeding equipment, even if she intends never to offer her baby a bottle. She should be shown how 'top and tail' her baby, and how to put on a leak-proof nappy. Useful hints can be passed on during a demonstration of how to bath a baby. It is extremely helpful for new mothers to know how to differentiate between minor and serious illness in a new baby, and she should know how to get expert help and advice quickly. Most mothers will have acquired a book on baby-care, but if asked, the midwife should be able to recommend a reliable, inexpensive one.

PHYSIOLOGICAL CHANGES

Forty-eight hours following delivery

Circulatory and renal systems   The increased blood volume manufactured to cope with pregnancy has largely been excreted by 48 hours. A massive diuresis commences soon after delivery, and the woman passes large amounts of urine. Blood volume may also have been reduced by blood loss at delivery, and the circulatory equilibrium will gradually be restored.

Endocrine system The physiological changes of pregnancy occur and are maintained under the influence of progesterone, and progesterone levels have fallen almost to pre-pregnancy levels by this time.

As lactation becomes established, prolactin levels rise; this change is 'permitted' by the falling progesterone and oestrogen levels.

The uterus The firmly contracted uterus immediately after delivery lies at about the level of the umbilicus. During the next 10 to 12 days, it will involute, that is, revert to its pre-pregnancy appearance, though it will usually be slightly more bulky. Involution occurs by means of a combination of muscular contraction and retraction, which means that the myometrium contracts but does not relax, and also by autolysis (that is, the cells of the myometrium are broken down and reabsorbed).

The lochia This is a plural word, referring to the blood loss from the placental site. It is still like a heavy period on the second day, and is red. As the placental site shrinks, so the lochia should become less.

The breasts The primipara is still secreting colostrum, but the multigravida will probably be lactating by this time. The colloquial expression is that the milk 'comes in'. The breasts then are full and heavy, with engorged veins standing out. The nipples may be shiny and slightly oedematous, and the baby may have temporary difficulty 'fixing'. With appropriate help this stage should soon pass.

Six weeks following delivery

By this time the woman's body has returned to a state similar to that before her pregnancy.

The renal and circulatory systems The progesterone effect of making the ureters tortuous and dilated has disappeared. The circulating volume has been normal for some time, and the haemoglobin should have returned to normal, with medical treatment if necessary.

The endocrine system If the woman is not breast-feeding, all hormone levels will have returned to normal, though the woman may not yet have ovulated and recommenced her periods. If she is breast-feeding, she will have high levels of prolactin, and will also be secreting oxytocin.

The uterus This will have involuted back almost to its pre-pregnancy size, though will always be slightly more bulky. The cervix, which was patulous and slightly open following delivery, will have closed, though a multiparous os is always slightly open, compared with the tightly closed nulliparous os.

The lochia The placental site should have shrunk and healed by this time, and the lochia should have ceased, having passed through the stages of being bright red, dark red, brown, yellowish white, and finally just a slight whitish vaginal discharge.

The breasts Although the breasts are now secreting more milk than they did at 48 hours, they will not now be tense, with the appearance of being over-full. They are still enlarged, but should not cause the mother undue discomfort.

PHYSICAL WELL-BEING

The midwife is required to visit the newly delivered mother, and to assess her physical and mental well-being. Because of all the physiological changes already described, it is usual to examine the woman systematically, in order to detect any problems, and to offer advice.

The midwife should approach the woman in a friendly, informal way, and enquire after her general well-being. The midwife wishes to find out if the mother is getting enough rest, if she is sleeping well, how she feels emotionally, and how she feels she is coping with, and relating to, the baby. Women often feel that the baby is the focus of attention, even though the woman herself has had to endure the pregnancy and labour (and most women feel a real sense of achievement afterwards). They will therefore appreciate someone taking the time to talk to them about how they are, provided that person has a real concern for them. It is then that anxieties may be shared and allayed; there are often feelings and fears, quite normal, which woman feel diffident to share, and about which they may feel vaguely guilty. After this the midwife proceeds to a physical examination.

The breasts These may be full and uncomfortable in the first few days, and the midwife gives help and advice with this. She looks for signs of infection, and if these appear, obtains medical advice immediately. If there are some difficulties with breast-feeding, ideally the midwife needs to be available when feeds are due, to give help and advice.

The uterus Involution is assessed daily by gentle palpation of the uterine fundus. The uterus should involute at a steady rate, until it is no longer palpable above the pubic symphysis at about 10 to 12 days.

The lochia   The pads should be inspected, to determine the colour and amount of lochia. The lochia should not be offensive, nor should blood clots or fragments of membrane be seen. The woman should be asked to inform the midwife if any of these abnormalities occur.

The perineum   This should be inspected, using a good light. Any tears, sutured or not, should be healing and clean. Initially the perineum may become very bruised and oedematous, and the midwife may need to refer the woman for ultrasound treatment, if this is available; regular analgesia is essential, and ice packs and regular use of the bath, shower or bidet will help.

Micturition   The woman should be passing good amounts of urine without difficulty, and the midwife must question her carefully to ascertain that this is so.

Bowels   The woman with a sutured perineum will dread her first bowel action, and may hold back from allowing it to happen. This problem must be detected promptly, and increasing fibre and fluids may be sufficient to give a well-formed stool, which may be passed without undue difficulty. If gentle aperients or bulking agents are needed, these should be given as necessary. Increasing the fruit intake too much does seem to upset some breast-fed babies, and mothers need to find out for themselves how much, and which fruits they can eat.

The legs   The relatively incompetent valves in the veins of the legs, together with the relative haemo-concentration, tend to predispose to thrombophlebitis, so the legs are examined for tenderness each day.

Rest and diet   Some women find it difficult to rest during the first few days following delivery. They are often very elated, but also have difficulty in finding opportunities to rest. However, it is very important that they should do so, and the midwife should encourage this. The woman should be encouraged to take adequate fibre in her diet, in order to re-establish good bowel habits. She needs plenty of fluid plus extra calories to make milk, if she is breast-feeding. If she normally eats a well-balanced diet, containing protein, carbohydrate and fats, she probably does not need to modify it. This is certainly not the time for drastic weight reducing diets, but the woman may be very receptive to general health education regarding reducing sugar and increasing fibre intake.

POSTNATAL EXERCISES

These are often taught by the physiotherapist, but the midwife should feel confident to teach them herself when necessary. She should certainly know what women have been taught, so that she can reinforce this teaching.

The aim of postnatal exercises is to strengthen the pelvic floor, and restore muscle tone. Failure to do this may lead to gynaecological problems such as stress incontinence and uterine prolapse often in later life.

THE POSTNATAL EXAMINATION

The woman has a final physical examination before leaving hospital. This is usually performed by the doctor, but there is no reason why it should not be performed by the midwife.

As well as checking all the items described above,

a tactful enquiry should be made as to the planned method of contraception. Every woman needs a break between babies, in order to recover fully, and so that she can give each one individual care and attention. Ovulation may recur at any time during the next few months, and it is quite possible for the woman to conceive again before she has had her first period. Breast-feeding certainly inhibits ovulation to some extent, but only women who are fully breast-feeding, that is, without giving even the occasional bottle, and feeding at frequent intervals, are reasonably well protected. If the breast feeding mother wishes to take the contraceptive pill, it is usual to give a 'progesterone-only' pill, because the woman already has a degree of protection, and because this type of pill will not have an adverse effect on lactation.

The woman is advised to visit her general practitioner six weeks after delivery for the six weeks postnatal check, or is given an appointment to return to the hospital if preferred. Hospital postnatal clinics tend now to cater mostly for those women who had some kind of obstetric or medical problem.

CARE IN THE COMMUNITY

On discharge from hospital, the mother and her new baby return to the care of the primary health care team. Those directly involved are the community midwife, the general practitioner and then the health visitor.

The community midwife visits the mother and baby until at least the 14th day, but may continue till the 28th day, after which she hands over their care to the health visitor.

The health visitor is a registered nurse who has completed a one-year course with particular emphasis on preventive aspects of health care for the whole community. She has a particular interest in the pre-school child, and should always be available to parents in an advisory capacity. She runs child health clinics, and also visits families at home. Many health visitors are 'GP attached' and so work closely with particular general practitioners.

FURTHER READING

BALL, J. A. & STANLEY, J. (1984) Stress and the mother, *Midwives Chronicle*, November.

LARYEA, M. (1984) *Postnatal Care—the Midwife's Role*. Edinburgh: Churchill Livingstone.

MATERNITY SERVICES ADVISORY COMMITTEE (1985) *Maternity Care in Action (Part III—Postnatal Care)*. London: HMSO.

ROBINSON, S. & THOMSON, A. M. (Eds.) (1988) *Midwives, Research and Childbirth*, Vol. 1. London: Chapman and Hall.

SWEET, B. (1982) *Mayes' Midwifery—a Textbook for Midwives*. London: Baillière Tindall.

15

PROBLEMS IN THE PUERPERIUM

INFECTION

Urinary tract infection

Urinary tract infection is common in the puerperium. If the woman suffered from such infection in the ante-natal period, it is likely to recur. If she has a degree of trauma to the urethra and a sore perineum the woman may not empty her bladder completely; urinary stasis will then lead to infection. The commonest causative organism is *Escherichia coli*. The woman is encouraged to drink as much as possible, a mid-stream specimen of urine is sent to the laboratory for culture, and the appropriate antibiotic is prescribed.

Uterine infection

The uterus is an excellent site for bacterial growth, and this may occur unless strict hygiene is observed, both by the woman, and those caring for her in labour.

The woman will have a pyrexia, often on about the third or fourth day following delivery. She will com-plain of malaise, and the uterus will feel bulky and may be tender. The lochia may be offensive.

A high vaginal swab is sent to the laboratory for culture, and the appropriate antibiotic prescribed. The woman is encouraged to rest, and to drink as much as she can.

Uterine infection may be caused by retained products of conception.

It is important that uterine infection is treated promptly and effectively, as it may lead to generalized pelvic infection with the possibility of salpingo-oophoritis, causing infertility.

Mastitis

Mastitis may occur at any time during lactation. Infection usually enters through minute cracks on the nipple. The breast will be tender over the infected section, and a wedge-shaped, red area appears. It is not necessary to stop breast-feeding unless there is a purulent discharge from the nipple; again, the appropriate antibiotic is commenced, when the causative organism has been identified from a specimen of milk sent to the laboratory. The woman usually feels extremely unwell, complaining of 'flu-like' symptoms, and pain in the breast.

If mastitis is not treated promptly, it may lead to breast abscess, requiring surgical incision.

BLEEDING

Primary postpartum haemorrhage

This is discussed in Chapter 12—'Abnormal Labour'. If associated with retained products of conception, these are evacuated under anaesthetic.

Secondary postpartum haemorrhage

This may occur at any time in the puerperium, and is usually associated with uterine infection and retained products of conception (see page 176).

The woman is often admitted to a gynaecological ward, rather than to the maternity unit, and ideally the baby should be admitted with her. The mother may then continue breast-feeding, and does not have the anxiety of being separated from her baby.

Retained products of conception

Any retained products of conception are evacuated under anaesthetic. This is done with great care, since it is relatively easy to perforate the uterus in the postnatal period.

PSYCHIATRIC COMPLICATIONS

'Third day blues'

Most mothers report feeling some degree of the 'blues' on or around the third day following delivery. They may feel 'weepy', bursting into tears for no good reason, or they may just feel withdrawn, and wish to be left alone. Part of the reason for this may be the passing of the feeling of elation and achievement which accompanies delivery for most women. Some women may feel that they have done all the hard work in producing the baby, but that the baby is receiving all the attention. The sensitive nurse will focus attention and concern on the mother. Women are often extremely tired at this stage following delivery, and this will not be conducive to a healthy mental state. Perineal bruising and swelling is likely to be at its worst, and the breasts are often full and uncomfortable. Hormones almost certainly play a part in the situation. 'Third day blues', then, are not considered abnormal, but it is most important to recognize when this situation exceeds normal limits, and becomes postnatal depression.

Postnatal depression

Postnatal depression becomes recognizable after about the fifth day following delivery, but may occur at any time during the baby's first year of life. When the onset is later, questioning may reveal that the woman has been suffering from a subclinical form of depression, but one more stressor, even a minor one, may precipitate an overt manifestation. For those who know the woman well, it is usually associated with some degree of personality change, and so there is an obvious advantage for the midwife who has been able to form a relationship with the woman during her pregnancy, and care for her throughout.

The woman will be 'weepy', crying for no apparent reason, and she will often manifest the typical features of depression—feelings of failure and worthlessness. Her sleep pattern will be disturbed, with early morning wakening; she will complain of feeling tired. She may start to neglect her appearance, the housework, and finally the baby. She will often feel that she has never related satisfactorily with the baby. This may be associated with unrealistic expectations of the baby and of motherhood.

The woman suffering from postnatal depression needs psychiatric treatment, close surveillance, and much support and understanding. Ideally this should come from the family, who must be helped to understand and accept the situation. The health visitor will be involved in the woman's care, and the community psychiatric nurse may also give support. Postnatal support groups, which may be run by organizations such as the local National Childbirth Trust group, or may be autonomous, provide a great deal of sympathetic help, but the depressed woman may find it extremely difficult to make the first contact, and to overcome the hurdle of attending the first meeting. Such groups are run by women who have experienced postnatal depression themselves, and so they are able to encourage sufferers that they may expect to recover completely.

Puerperal psychosis

This a much less common complication. The woman demonstrates definite, and often bizarre, personality changes. The psychotic manifestations may include delusions, hallucinations, and hearing voices, and there is a danger that the woman may harm herself or her baby. Ideally again the mother and baby are admitted to hospital together. Treatment is long-term.

THROMBOEMBOLIC DISORDERS

Superficial venous thrombosis

The newly delivered mother is particularly prone to superficial venous thrombosis because of the pro-gesterone effects on the veins of the legs, and the changes in blood chemistry brought about by preg-nancy which cause the blood to coagulate rather more readily than in the non-pregnant state. Progesterone relaxes plain muscle, so that the leg veins are dilated, causing relative incompetence of the valves, and slug-gish venous return. Women suffering from varicose veins are particularly prone to such complications.

Preventive measures include early ambulation, par-ticularly after caesarean section, the use of support stockings, or anti-embolic 'TED' stockings, and the teaching and supervision of leg exercises.

The main symptom of thrombophlebitis is tender-ness over the affected area of the vein.

Deep vein thrombosis

When a thrombus occurs in one of the deep veins of the leg, it is treated with anticoagulant therapy.

Signs and symptoms usually include a low-grade pyrexia and tenderness over the thrombus, but the diagnosis is only confirmed on ultrasound scan or venography.

Women with a history of thromboembolic disorders are prone to recurrence, and may receive anticoagulant therapy as a prophylactic measure. This requires careful administration and supervision during pregnancy and following delivery. It is usual to give heparin during pregnancy, but other anticoagulants may be used following delivery, though these are prescribed with caution if the woman is breast-feeding.

Pulmonary embolus

If a thrombus is present in the deep femoral or pelvic veins, there is a significant risk of pulmonary embolus. This is one of the commoner causes of maternal death in the UK.

HELPING PARENTS COPE WITH GRIEF

Because public expectations of the maternity services are high, it can be a devastating experience for all concerned if a pregnancy does not have a successful conclusion. Many parents expect nothing less than a perfect baby, with the sophistication of antenatal investigations today. However, unexplained stillbirths still occur, and unexpected congenital abnormalities do present themselves. This is partly because not all abnormalities may be detected by antenatal screening.

Congenital abnormality

This is discussed in Chapter 18—'The Baby with Special Needs'. Parents who produce an abnormal baby experience a variety of emotions, including grieving for the normal, healthy baby they had expected to produce. One or both parents may reject the baby, and patient, sensitive support is required.

The recognized features of the grief process include denial and a feeling of numbness, then anger and a tendency to direct the blame at some other person or a mechanical cause, followed by sadness and expression of grief.

Initially parents will have a limited ability to absorb and accept the situation, and must be given new information as they are able to cope with it. It may be months before they appreciate the long-term implications for their future as a family, particularly if the baby is severely handicapped.

Once again, support groups comprising parents who have similar problems may be an excellent source of emotional and practical help.

When a baby is born with a condition such as spina bifida the whole situation must be assessed. Sometimes it is felt appropriate to treat such a baby actively; on other occasions it may seem best to give loving care, and allow nature to take its course. Medical staff will attempt to give parents a fair, overall view of the situation and prognosis, should support their decision, and respect their wishes. Making such a decision places the family in an agonizing position.

Stillbirth and neonatal death

Caring for parents who know their baby will be stillborn is very demanding of staff.

In the past midwives and doctors often pretended

that the problem did not exist, and made no reference to the fact that the baby had died. As in any grief situation, parents prefer openness and the opportunity to express their own feelings. Their wishes for care in labour should be discussed, and respected as far as possible. The midwife will talk to the parents about their feelings about seeing and cuddling the baby after delivery. No pressure is brought to bear, and many parents finally decide to hold their child. A photograph is usually taken, and is placed in the mother's notes if the parents do not wish to have it at the time. Many parents request such a picture after a period of time.

Parents whose baby is dying also need much help and support.

The mother's wishes regarding her immediate post-natal care should be discussed and respected. Some women wish to be alone, while others prefer the company of other women. For many women, early transfer home is the ideal solution, provided they have sympathetic help and support.

Arranging a funeral is expensive for young parents, and the Death Grant is a nominal sum. A less expensive funeral may be arranged through the hospital authorities, but parents are often distressed at the idea of an unmarked grave. Such arrangements must be discussed with tact and sympathy.

FURTHER READING

BEREZIN, N. (1982) *After a Loss in Pregnancy*. New York: Simon and Schuster.

COX, J. L. (1986) *Postnatal Depression*. Edinburgh: Churchill Livingstone.

KOHNER, N. (1985) *Midwives and Stillbirth* (Report on a Joint Workshop—Royal College of Midwives and Health Education Council). London: Health Education Council.

LLEWELLYN-JONES, D. (1982) *Fundamentals of Obstetrics and Gynaecology*, Vol. I, 3rd edn. London: Faber & Faber.

MURRAY PARKES, C. (1986) *Bereavement*. London: Tavistock Publications.

SWEET, B. R. (1988) *Mayes' Midwifery—a Textbook for Midwives*, 11th edn. London: Baillière Tindall.

16

THE NORMAL BABY

CHARACTERISTICS AND APPEARANCE

The newborn human baby is a complex, highly aware being, contrary to popular belief.

The special senses

Sight Experiments and observation have shown that the newborn baby can see quite clearly over a short distance, and there was no fault in the design which decreed that he should focus clearly on a point approximately 20 cm away from him. This, of course, enables him to see his mother's face clearly from the feeding position. He is able to fix and follow visually through a limited field objects which interest him, though his attention span is short, but babies have been shown to find faces the most interesting. They also prefer bright colours.

Hearing The baby responds to sound; he will startle at sudden, loud noises, but will often settle in response to a gentle speaking or singing voice or rhythmic music. A female voice is preferred. Crying babies will often settle to the sound of a vacuum cleaner, for example, and tapes of soothing music have been produced in recent years. The uterus is, of course, not a silent environment, with the maternal heart beat and bowel sounds being quite loud from within, as well as external sound effects, and these tapes reproduce the rhythms of a heart beating. Babies *in utero* have also appeared to show preferences for different kinds of music by reacting differently.

Smell   It has been demonstrated that a baby recognizes the distinctive smell of his mother within a few days of birth, and will turn his head towards a breast pad soaked in her milk, rather than that of another woman.

Taste   A baby will certainly grimace if given something which tastes unpleasant, and will spit it out.

Touch   Newborn babies relax and settle if stroked and caressed; they prefer to be held firmly and securely, and will often cry if an uncertain adult is handling them.

Reflex responses

The normal newborn baby has a repertoire of neurological responses which may be elicited.

The Moro or 'startle' reflex   The stimulus of a sudden loud noise or movement will make the baby move his arms and legs in a characteristic fashion.

The rooting reflex   When the breast, or anything soft and warm, such as a blanket, is felt on the cheek, the baby will turn his head in that direction and search for the nipple.

The sucking reflex   This is stimulated by the presence of a teat or the nipple in the mouth.

The 'walking' or 'stepping' reflex   When the baby is held upright, and the plantar surface of the foot put in contact with a hard surface, such as the edge of a table, the baby will make stepping movements. The purpose of this reflex is still unclear, and it disappears within weeks, but its absence would arouse suspicions of some neurological deficit.

The grasp reflex   The baby will close his fingers tightly over any object placed in the palm of his hand. He does not learn to release objects deliberately until he is several months old.

It is important for the nurse to appreciate how much a new baby can do, and how aware he is of his surroundings, so that she may help the new mother to observe her baby, obtain pleasure from his responses, and be aware if all is not well. If a mother feels she has a response from her baby, she tends to feel rewarded for all the hard work involved, and will stimulate her baby more, so that there is good interaction between them, and the start of a good relationship.

The average birth weight for a Caucasian baby is around 3.5 kg, and his length 50–52 cm.

He will be rounded and pink; he lies with limbs flexed, and responds to stimuli. He may not cry at birth, if delivery has been normal, and calmly conducted; this often worries the new parents, but the midwife's main concern is that the baby should establish spontaneous respiration immediately, and become pink. The parents may then be reassured. The baby will often be very alert and wide awake for about an hour after birth, and during this time should have an undisturbed time with his parents and be put to the breast if his mother wishes to breast-feed. This is thought to be a very important period of time for the new family, when parent/child attachment develops in a significant way.

NEEDS

Like any other human being the new baby has both physical and emotional needs.

Physical needs

Warmth   The baby needs a warm environment, since he is not able to adjust to changes in temperature very efficiently.

Food and fluid   He needs the correct amount of fluid and calories, provided by breast milk or one of the modified baby milks.

Hygiene   The new baby is very susceptible to infection and scrupulous cleanliness is vital.

Emotional needs

Love and security   The baby is sensitive to his environment and needs physical contact, stimulation and the security of a settled routine, though this may take some time to establish.

DAILY OBSERVATIONS

While mother and baby are in the care of the midwife, usually for 14 days, it is usual to check the baby each day. In the process of adapting to extrauterine life, babies often acquire minor infections, and these must be treated promptly to avoid complications.

General appearance   Following the alert period immediately after birth, the baby may become sleepy for a couple of days, particularly if his mother has received a significant amount of pethidine for pain relief in labour. However, a baby who is sleepy and lethargic after this time needs careful observation and perhaps medical investigation, so the baby's general appearance is noted. He should be active when fully awake, and lies with his limbs flexed. His colour should be pink. He should demand his feeds, should feed well, and then settle, even if he does not sleep. The mother should be encouraged to voice any uncertainties during discussion on feeding and settling.

After noting the baby's general appearance, it is useful to examine the baby briefly but systematically.

The eyes   These are checked for the presence of any discharge.

The mouth   This is checked for the presence of thrush, which looks like milk curds.

The umbilical cord   This should be cleaned using a spirit swab whenever necessary, and often hexachlorophane powder is applied as well. Many mothers are afraid to touch the cord, and need help and encouragement. If kept clean and dry, the cord should separate in about four to five days, though a thick one will take longer. The plastic cord clamp placed on the cord at delivery is usually removed after two to three days. The umbilicus may become 'sticky', offensive and red, indicating infection, and this must be treated promptly.

The skin   The skin, and particularly the skin folds and the napkin area, are checked for spots or soreness.

Identification   In hospital it is important to prevent the distress caused by handing a mother the wrong baby, or of allowing the possibility of her suspecting that this may have happened. Most maternity units have strict policies about identity labels for mothers and babies, and it is wise, when checking the baby each day, to check that he is wearing at least one, and preferably two, identity bands.

SCREENING

All new babies are screened for certain conditions in the neonatal period. This is discussed in more detail in Chapter 19—'Social Aspects'.

MINOR PROBLEMS

The common minor problems have already been mentioned in describing the daily examination of the baby.

Minor infections

'Sticky' eyes   Even a watery discharge from the eyes must be observed carefully. The eye is swabbed gently every four hours or at feed times. In hospital this is done with sterile normal saline and sterile cotton wool balls. At home the mother may use cooled boiled water. Any purulent or persistent discharge must be investigated and treated, using antibiotic drops or ointment.

Septic spots   Most new babies develop some spots, but these must be treated promptly if there is any sign of infection.

Paronychia   The baby may occasionally develop infection alongside the fingernail.

Thrush This may occur in bottle- or breast-fed babies, and is common if the mother has had vaginal candidiasis (moniliasis). It is usually seen first in the baby's mouth, as whitish patches, looking like milk, but which cannot be scraped gently away. It often passes through the digestive tract, and causes red, sore buttocks. It is treated with oral nystatin, given after feeds, and nystatin cream is applied to the buttocks, preferably with the buttocks exposed to the air.

Sore buttocks

This is a common problem, frequently caused by inadequate cleaning of the buttocks at nappy changes, or by infrequent nappy changing. Once mother and baby are at home, it may be due to nappy hygiene, if terry nappies are used. Tactful questioning about the washing powder used or the number of rinses given may give a clue as to the cause. If she is using disposable nappies, the mother may need to try different brands. Important points in subsequent prevention are:

Thorough washing of the whole nappy area at each change.
Use of a good barrier agent, such as zinc and castor oil cream.
Use of a 'one way' nappy liner or one of the newer brands of disposable nappy which are designed to prevent urine remaining against the skin.
Changing the nappy as soon as it is wet or dirty.
Thorough sanitization of nappies, either using the proprietary hypochlorite solutions or by boiling (by machine or hand, though the latter is now old fashioned).
Thorough washing and rinsing of nappies using a soap or non-biological powder. The use of fabric

conditioner may result in skin irritation on some babies.

Leaving off the plastic pants for a time each day, or better still, leaving the baby without a nappy for a time each day (having taken suitable precautions!)

Jaundice

The jaundice seen in newborn babies is called physiological jaundice.

The fetus has a high level of haemoglobin, and therefore red cells, to enable him to perform adequate gaseous exchange via the placenta. Once he is born, and his lungs are functioning, this higher level of haemoglobin is no longer necessary. One of the breakdown products of haemoglobin is bilirubin, and as the liver cannot excrete it all immediately, most babies have a degree of jaundice, though it is not always noticeable.

This circulating bilirubin is fat-soluble, rather than water-soluble, and cannot be excreted by the kidneys until it is water-soluble. The process of converting bilirubin from a fat-soluble to a water-soluble state is called 'conjugation'. Ultraviolet light speeds up this process, hence the use of phototherapy. The baby is nursed in an incubator, under a special light source.

Nursing needs for baby and mother include the following.

The eyes   The eyes are protected by the use of fabric goggles, which may be held in place by elastic bandage, such as 'Netelast'.

Comfort   He is nursed naked for maximum effect, but some babies seem to feel insecure, having just got used to clothes, and will not settle. This will add to the mother's distress; she may feel very anxious about lifting her seemingly fragile infant out of the incubator, and will need sensitive support and reassurance, as well as some practical help.

Extra fluids The baby should have extra fluid—
opinion varies as to whether this should be milk or
boiled water, but the baby loses more fluid by evap-
oration, and he may have loose stools as well, so this
fluid must be replaced. The jaundiced baby may be
sleepy and slow to feed, however, so it may not be
easy to give him extra.

If jaundice is very marked, the serum bilirubin levels
are measured regularly, until they begin to fall. Occasionally brain damage may occur as a result of high
levels of unconjugated bilirubin circulating, and so it
may be necessary to measure the ratio of unconjugated
and conjugated bilirubin.

If neonatal jaundice is caused by any other condition,
it is called pathological jaundice. It may be due to:

Rhesus or ABO incompatibility.
Breast milk—occasionally the mother's breast milk
may contain substances which inhibit conjugation
of bilirubin.
Infection—certain infections may lead to haemolysis
of red cells.
Obstructive jaundice—occasionally there may be a
congenital anomaly of the biliary tract.

High serum bilirubin levels may necessitate exchange transfusion, when measured quantities of the
baby's blood are removed, and replaced by donor
blood.

HYGIENE

Baby bathing has been rather a ritual for most of the
20th century, but is not a daily necessity in the early
days as long as the baby's face, bottom and skin folds
are carefully washed and dried daily.

This is often called 'topping and tailing'. Mothers are taught to do this soon after delivery. The baby is less likely to become chilled during this procedure, even if the new mother is rather slow, as she can be shown how to do it without undressing the baby completely.

Babies are no longer bathed following delivery, largely because of the risk of chilling. It is common practice not to bath the baby until the cord has separated, though this does not have to be a strict rule.

Mothers usually want to be shown how to bath their babies. It is most helpful to offer practical suggestions and teach principles.

Principles include the following:

The room should be warm and draught-free.
Everything should be ready beforehand, with clean clothes warming on a radiator if possible, and everything within easy reach of the mother.
The bath, and the mother's chair, should be at a comfortable height.
The baby's face and head should be washed before removing the nappy.
The whole process should be completed as quickly as possible while the baby is small, though later it will become fun for all concerned!

In all such teaching, the emphasis should be on practicality, and mothers encouraged to find the best way for themselves. For example, some women will feel happiest bathing and changing the baby on a changing mat on the floor; as long as there is no draught and conditions are reasonably clean, there is no reason why they should not do so. The baby will fit into the conventional type of baby bath for a relatively short time, and carrying the bath full of water is awkward, as well as hazardous for the mother's back. There are various alternatives, such as a washing up bowl, or a baby bath which fits over the family bath, which may be preferred. The use of a baby bathing solution in the water speeds up the process and will minimize the risk of chilling.

FURTHER READING

ILLINGWORTH, R. S. (1975) *The Normal Child*, 6th edn. Edinburgh: Churchill Livingstone.

KEAY, A. J. & MORGAN, D. M. (1978) *Craig's Care of the Newly Born Infant*, 6th edn. Edinburgh: Churchill Livingstone.

MCFARLANE, A. (1977) *The Psychology of Childbirth*. London: Fontana.

SWEET, B. R. (1988) *Mayes' Midwifery—a Textbook for Midwives*, 11th edn. London: Baillière Tindall.

17

INFANT FEEDING

The aims of infant feeding are to give the baby an adequate fluid intake and the necessary balance of protein, fat and carbohydrate, plus vitamins and minerals. The baby has very special metabolic needs, and the only food which will meet his needs exactly is his own mother's milk. Despite ever increasing knowledge, the finest scientific research, and competition for the market, modified cows' milk does not equate to human breast milk.

THE METHOD OF FEEDING

The factors which influence mothers in this matter are many and varied. Fashions change, and breast- and bottle-feeding alternate in popularity over the years. Attitudes within the woman's family are very important, as is the attitude of her partner. Her circumstances may influence her decision very strongly; if she has no privacy, or needs to return to work as quickly as possible because of financial constraints, she is more likely to opt for artificial feeding. Some women feel very shy about exposing and handling their breasts, and often find the idea of breast-feeding quite repulsive. The breasts, in Western society, are seen as sexual objects, not as feeding apparatus, and the woman's partner may feel jealous of the baby's use of them. The latter two reasons are often not discussed openly, and the real reasons may be hidden behind such explanations as wishing to share the feeding role or wanting to be free to go out. On the other hand, women may feel strongly that breast-feeding is best for the baby, and because it is the natural way to feed, be firmly committed to the idea.

The role of the nurse or midwife is to help each mother, if she requires such help, to make the right decision for her. Breast-feeding should certainly be encouraged, but the reluctant or less than fully committed breast-feeder will rarely succeed. Women who feed their babies artifically should not be made to feel guilty in any way, but should be supported in the decision they have made.

It has been traditional to list the advantages and disadvantages of breast-feeding. Certainly the breast-fed baby enjoys close contact with his mother, but the mother who is bottle-feeding should be encouraged to cuddle her baby, and interact with him as she feeds him. There is no reason why they cannot have skin-to-skin contact if she wishes. Traditionally breast-feeding has been said to be expensive, because the woman requires a better diet. Most women enjoy a reasonable standard of nutrition, and although she certainly needs to increase both her fluid and calorific intake, the breast-feeding mother who already eats a healthy diet will not need to make drastic changes in her eating habits. Artificial feeding requires financial outlay for sterilizing equipment and solution or tablets (though the container may be improvised, as long as the solution is made up accurately). Unless the mother is receiving Social Security benefits, and is eligible for free milk for her baby, she has to consider the expense of buying milk. Establishing breast-feeding can be a time-consuming, demanding process for some mothers, but once this initial period has passed, it is quicker and easier. Unfortunately, despite professional and consumer voices being raised in support of breast-feeding, breast-feeding in public tends to cause shocked and embarrassed reactions. Few stores provide mothers' rooms, and so the breast-feeding woman may encounter real difficulties when she is out. However, if she gives careful thought to her clothing, she should be able to feed unobtrusively, and avoid causing offence.

The unquestioned benefit conferred by breast-feeding is the passing of antibodies to the baby. He will thus acquire immunity to any disease to which his mother is immune, which is effective until his own immune responses mature. This may have a bearing on the fact that 'sudden infant death syndrome' (SIDS or 'cot death') is seen significantly less often in breast-fed babies. There are also certain anti-infective factors in breast milk, protecting the breast-fed baby from a variety of organisms. Thus the breast-fed baby is doubly protected, since his feed is not liable to contamination and bacterial growth in the same way as that of the bottle-fed baby. Cows' milk allergy has received a great deal of attention in the past few years, and the baby who is breast-fed for the first six months is less likely to suffer from this.

In the past few years attention has also been drawn to the dangers of inaccurate mixing of feeds. Baby milk formulae have been further modified since the days when babies became extremely ill with hypernatraemia (high sodium level), but it is still very important that mothers appreciate the need to mix feeds exactly as instructed on the packet. Artificially fed babies gain weight more quickly, and it has been thought that excessive weight gain in infancy contributes to obesity and associated ill health in later life. It is currently advised that mixed feeding be commenced as late as possible, and not before four months. However, the temptation to thicken the bottle feed with a rusk or cereal is not always resisted, particularly in the interests of giving the parents an undisturbed night's sleep.

THE PRINCIPLES OF INFANT FEEDING

The giving of unmodified cows' milk to a baby under the age of six months is a dangerous practice, and is definitely contraindicated.

This can be appreciated if the constituents of human and cows' milk are compared (Table 17.1). It is also interesting to note the constitution of colostrum, the substance secreted by the breasts for the first two to three days, to meet the newborn baby's dietary needs.

It is no longer considered appropriate to feed babies by a rigid schedule, and all healthy full-term babies may be fed on demand. A routine will usually emerge for demand feeding so that home life can be ordered within a few weeks.

Each baby is an individual, just as his mother is, and so guidelines as to fluid and calorific requirements should only be regarded as average figures.

A newborn baby requires 150–165 ml of fluid per kg of body weight per day. This amount is not given at birth, just as the breast-fed baby does not receive large quantities of milk immediately. A typical plan might be to give:

Day 1–60 ml per kg of body weight in 24 hours
Day 2–60 ml per kg of body weight in 24 hours

Table 17.1 Comparison of contents of colostrum, breast milk and cows' milk

Constituent	Colostrum	Human milk	Cows' milk
Protein	8%	1.5%	3.5%
Sugar	3.5%	7%	4.5%
Fat	2.5%	3.5%	3.5%
Minerals	0.4%	0.2%	0.7%
Water	85.6%	87.8%	87.8%

Day 3–90 ml per kg of body weight in 24 hours
Day 4–120 ml per kg of body weight in 24 hours
Day 5–150 ml per kg of body weight in 24 hours

If a baby is alert and attentive when awake, settles and sleeps well, and gains weight steadily, then he is considered to be thriving. Breast-feeding mothers often become anxious because they cannot measure the baby's intake as do bottle-feeding mothers, and this anxiety makes many give up breast-feeding. However, guidelines such as these may be given to reassure the worried mother.

A great deal of importance is attached to the 'percentile' chart when growth and development is being monitored. A percentile chart is based on observations of a particular group of babies and children, and lines running across the graph-type chart give the 10th, 50th and 90th 'centiles'. This means that at any given age the weight of 10% of the population will fall below the line which indicates the 10th centile. Similarly, 10% of the population will have a weight above that of the 90th centile (in other words, 90% of the population would fall below that line). Birth weight is plotted on the percentile chart, and the baby is then expected to gain weight, and to grow in length and head circumference, within these parameters.

BREAST-FEEDING

Establishing breast-feeding

As already mentioned, this may be a difficult time for some mothers. Probably the biggest problem in this area is the giving of conflicting advice, which causes much anxiety and loss of confidence in new mothers. It is one of the greatest challenges facing the midwife involved in postnatal care.

Research has shown that the baby put to the breast as soon as possible after delivery is likely to breast-feed successfully after a shorter period. At this stage the baby is usually alert and active, and will readily root and suck. (See Chapter 16–'The Normal Baby'.)

The most important factor in successful breast-feeding is encouraging the baby to 'fix' correctly on the nipple. Failure to achieve this is the principal cause of all the classic breast problems—sore, cracked nipples, leading to breast infections, and much distress and anxiety.

It is difficult for the mother, from her angle, to see when the baby is correctly fixed, particularly if she has large breasts, and a sore perineum so that she has difficulty sitting comfortably and relaxing. She then needs guidance to help her recognize when it 'feels' right, and to position the baby and herself correctly.

The baby needs to take the whole nipple into his mouth, so that his lips are round the areola, and so that his gums place pressure on the areola (and therefore on the underlying milk ducts) rather than the end of the nipple (Fig. 17.1). The mother is shown how to look for the movement of the areola in and out of the baby's mouth as he sucks, which indicates that he has the nipple drawn out across his tongue, and is suckling successfully.

The breast-fed baby tends to need feeding more frequently than the artificially fed baby, particularly in the early days, and mothers need to be prepared for this. The more the baby feeds, the more quickly and successfully will the milk supply become established. For most women frequent feeding should not result in sore nipples if the baby fixes correctly. There is therefore little place for time limits and clock-watching, which were both fashionable until relatively recently.

There are two processes involved in establishing breast-feeding. One is milk production, and the other is milk 'let-down'. Milk may be produced successfully,

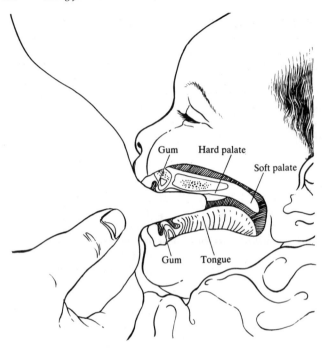

Fig. 17.1   A baby breast-feeding. Note that the nipple is well back in the baby's mouth.

but if it is not 'let down', it does not become easily available to the baby. When milk is secreted by the milk-producing cells, or acini, under the influence of prolactin from the anterior lobe of the pituitary gland, some of this milk passes into the ducts, and will be available at the start of the next feed. However, most of the milk remains in the cells, and is not released, or let down, until oxytocin is secreted by the posterior lobe of the pituitary gland. Oxytocin causes contraction of the acini, so that the milk passes into the ducts, and some will often spurt out from the nipple.

When the let down reflex is well established, it is frequently initiated by a stimulus such as the sound of the baby crying. The milk available to the baby at the start of the feed is called the 'foremilk', and the milk which is released on let-down is the 'hindmilk'. The hindmilk is more satisfying, containing more fat and therefore calories. If the baby does not have long enough at each breast, he will not be satisfied—another reason for abandoning the clock!

Feeding her baby becomes every mother's main preoccupation once she has delivered, and it is important that she leaves the care of the midwife feeling confident that she is able to do this.

Breast problems

Although correct fixing of the baby at the breast should reduce the incidence of breast problems, they will still be seen, and will cause much misery for some women. It is important that they are treated promptly and appropriately.

Sore nipples Some women experience pain within the nipple at the start of the feed, in the early days following delivery. This pain usually resolves as the baby sucks, provided he is well positioned. It becomes a problem if the mother becomes tense, so that her let-down reflex is inhibited, and the baby does not obtain the hindmilk. She needs explanation, reassurance, perhaps preventive analgesics before feeding is anticipated, and perhaps positive help with some relaxation techniques.

The more common problem is soreness of the nipple skin, which will look red, and will eventually become cracked. If the mother can be helped to start feeding, and get the baby well positioned, the soreness does not usually persist throughout the feed. Various creams and sprays have been fashionable, and mothers may feel they are helpful, but many feel they are not necessary. Rubbing a little expressed breast milk onto the nipple will help to heal cracks, and women should be advised to expose the nipples as much as possible. The 'Mexican hat' type of nipple shield fits closely over the nipple and gives good protection. Some midwives still advocate resting the nipple, but this does interfere with the establishment of feeding, and the problem is not truly resolved until the cause is rectified.

Cracked nipples   If a sore nipple has reached the stage of being cracked and bleeding, it does need to be rested, initially for 24 hours. It is then vitally important to help the mother position the baby well.

Flat or inverted nipples   With the best help in the world, flat or inverted nipples are prone to soreness, because the baby cannot draw the nipple out across his tongue as he sucks, and so will chew the nipple, rather than putting pressure on the areola with his gums and tongue. Nipples which do not protract well (see page 32) have adhesions within the nipple structure. These may be broken down to a certain extent in the antenatal period, by the use of 'Woolwich shells', which are worn inside the bra, so that the nipple protrudes through the hole, putting pressure on the area where the adhesions would be. Various manipulations, such as pulling and rolling the nipples may also be advised. Opinion is divided as to the usefulness of all these procedures, but they probably do no harm.

Full breasts   When the milk 'comes in' the breasts often become very full and tender. The areola is then likely to be tense and slightly oedematous, and the baby will have great difficulty fixing. Engorgement is an extreme over-fullness, where there is no milk flow at all initially. The woman is very uncomfortable, often holding her arms cautiously away from her sides. A milk flow must be established, unless it has arisen as a result of stopping breast-feeding. Stasis of milk within the breasts is likely to lead to infection. Alleviation of over-full breasts includes having a hot bath, to encourage leakage, or using hot flannels for the same purpose. Some milk is then expressed by hand, to relieve the tension in the areolae, and the baby is put to the breast. Frequent feeding is usually helpful. It is important to let the baby take all the available milk from one breast, and then to offer the other breast first at the next feed. This situation will usually resolve itself, as the breasts fill on a supply and demand basis. As time passes the breasts secrete more milk to meet the baby's greater needs as he grows, but accommodate it more comfortably. The breasts must be supported comfortably, with an old fashioned breast binder if necessary. The breasts will be so enlarged that the nursing bra may not adapt sufficiently to give the necessary support. Analgesics are given as required.

Blocked duct One milk duct may repeatedly fail to empty, and the breast over that area will become red, lumpy and painful. The mother may feel shivery and unwell, and this will readily lead to mastitis if the duct does not clear. Gentle massage of the painful area will help to clear the duct.

Mastitis When infection occurs in the breast the mother feels unwell, complaining of flu-like symptoms. The temperature and pulse rate will be raised. The breast is tender, with a wedge-shaped, red area over the infected lobe. A specimen of milk is sent to the laboratory for culture and sensitivity testing, and the appropriate antibiotic is prescribed. Temporary cessation of feeding from the infected side may or may not be advised, depending on the causative organism.

Breast abscess   This may result from mastitis being treated unsuccessfully or from delay in treatment. The baby is not fed from the infected breast. Surgical incision is often necessary.

ARTIFICIAL FEEDING

Although they do not equate to human breast milk, modern baby milks are formulated so as to be as similar in composition as possible. They therefore form a very good substitute. As well as being modified so that protein, fat and carbohydrate contents are similar to those in human milk, vitamins, minerals and trace elements are added.

Making up feeds

As already discussed, it is essential that feeds are made up accurately, following the instructions on the tin, and using the measuring scoop provided for the particular milk used. Modern milks mix easily; the powder is usually added to the boiled water in a wide-necked bottle, the bottle is capped, and shaken. Thus a minimum of equipment is used, so reducing the infection risk. Sugar is not added to baby milks. Feeds may be made up for 24 hours, and stored in the refrigerator.

Cartons of 'ready-to-feed' milk are now available over the counter.

Feeding technique

The feed is warmed if required (though babies in hospital are often fed milk at room temperature). This may be done by placing the bottle in a jug of hot water, which must be kept well away from toddlers to prevent accidental scalding. This is not done until the feed is about to be given. Heating babies' bottles in microwave ovens is not recommended, partly because of the danger of over-heating and partly because of changes occurring in the milk itself as a result of the microwave activity. The bottle remains capped whenever it is not in the baby's mouth. The mother checks the temperature of the feed, by shaking a little onto the inside of her wrist.

The baby is held comfortably, in the crook of the mother's arm, and the bottle tipped, so as to fill the neck of the bottle and the teat with milk, so that the body does not swallow air. Most babies will pause for breath at some point, and during a natural break, the baby should be supported in an upright position, to encourage him to burp. (This seems to be a British tradition, and some would question the necessity for it.)

Sterilization of equipment

It is essential that all feeding equipment is sterilized during the first nine to 12 months of the baby's life. After this time, when he is mobile, he will be rushing around on the floor, putting everything into his mouth, clean or not, and will be much more able to withstand infection.

The proprietary preparations available for sterilization of feeding equipment come in fluid or tablet form, and are all based on sodium hypochlorite or sodium dichloroisocyanurate. Various containers are available, but the container may be improvised, as long as the solution is diluted accurately. The solution is changed every 24 hours. Bottles, teats, spoons, dishes and dummies must be washed thoroughly, and rinsed in running water before being completely immersed in the sterilizing solution. Teats are rubbed with salt, inside and out, to remove any traces of milk curd. No metal objects should be immersed in sodium hypochlorite, so spoons must be plastic. It is very important to ensure that no air bubbles remain in bottles or teats, and teats in particular should not be allowed to float. The proprietary sterilizing units include a piece of plastic designed to prevent this. The best way to prevent air bubbles remaining in bottles is to use sufficient solution to allow upright storage.

The manufacturers now recommend that equipment should be rinsed in boiled water after removal from the sterilizing fluid.

All mothers, including those who intend to breast-feed fully, should be taught these simple principles before leaving the postnatal ward.

A recent innovation on the baby goods market is a steam sterilizer for feeding equipment.

FURTHER READING

KITZINGER, S. (1979) *The Experience of Breast Feeding*. London: Croom Helm.

ROBINSON, S. & THOMSON, A. M. (Eds.) (1988) Why don't women breast feed? In *Midwives, Research and Chilbirth*, Vol. 1. London: Chapman and Hall.

SCOWEN, P. & WELLS J. (Eds.) (1979) *Feeding Children in the First Year*. London: B. Edsall (for the Health Visitors' Association).

STANWAY, P. & STANWAY, A. (1978) *Breast is Best*. London: Pan Books.

18

THE BABY WITH SPECIAL NEEDS

The baby with special needs also has parents with special needs. Supporting families with an abnormal baby was discussed briefly in Chapter 15—'Problems in the Puerperium'. The family of a baby who is sick and needing special or intensive care also need much support.

The problems of mothers with babies in the Special Care Baby Unit are well documented and discussed. Awareness of these problems have led to changes in policy in such units, and attitudes are now much more open and flexible. The needs of the family have been taken into account, and in most units, older brothers and sisters are now welcomed, fathers are encouraged to help care for their babies, and the rest of the family are welcome to see the baby, though this may be from a viewing corridor if the baby is very sick. The mother is encouraged to visit the baby as soon as possible after delivery, and physical contact is thought to be very important for both. Even if the baby is too ill to be cuddled, parents are encouraged to put their hands into the incubator and touch and talk to the baby. As soon as possible, if they feel able, parents are involved in the baby's care. Medical staff should make themselves available to explain and discuss the baby's problems, treatment and prognosis. Parents may need such explanations repeatedly; having a sick baby is not the expected outcome of pregnancy in most cases, and is the exception. The new family have to cope with enquiries, questions and the anxiety of the rest of the family. They may feel they cannot go through the usual rituals surrounding birth, such as sending notification to family and friends, and placing an announcement in the newspaper.

THE LOW BIRTH WEIGHT BABY

Low birth weight is defined as a birth weight below 2.5 kilograms.

Very low birth weight is a recently introduced category; many more very small babies survive now, and, more importantly, grow into healthy children. Very low birth weight is defined as a birth weight below 1.5 kg.

The low birth weight baby may be small because he had been born before term, or he may be 'light for dates'. The two need to be differentiated, since they require different treatment. The baby who qualifies for both categories presents a more complex problem.

The preterm baby

Gestation and viability have been discussed in Chapter 6—'Normal Pregnancy'. Many babies born before 28 weeks now prove their viability by surviving intact (that is, to be fit and healthy) with improved neonatal intensive care.

The preterm baby is likely to encounter various problems and has certain specific needs during early life.

Nutrition Swallowing, cough and sucking reflexes will be immature, and the preterm baby may tire before he has taken enough feed to satisfy his nutritional needs. Tube feeding is often necessary, and this may be by nasogastric or orojejunal tube. The risk of gastric reflux and aspiration is less with the latter type. The preterm infant has greater calorific requirements, but may not absorb feeds efficiently.

Warmth The preterm infant has little 'brown fat', which is present in the infant at term and has important insulating properties. Heat loss occurs readily, and preterm infants are usually dressed in bonnets, bootees and mittens, and wear normal baby clothes whenever possible. (This latter also has a personalizing effect.) The Special Care Baby Unit is kept very warm. Body heat may be conserved by the use of a 'heat shield' made of Perspex; this is placed over the baby inside the incubator or cot. Heat loss uses up valuable resources, depleting glycogen stores, and rendering the baby even less capable of feeding well.

Protection from infection The preterm infant is poorly equipped to withstand infection, and unfortunately, the Special Care Baby Unit is particularly prone to invasion by virulent organisms found mostly in hospitals. Some of these are resistant to many of the antibiotics in current use, and this poses a problem. Measures such as strict hand washing, the wearing of gowns when handling babies, strict disinfection and sterilizing techniques, and the provision of individual equipment are generally practised.

Jaundice The preterm infant is likely to develop physiological jaundice because of his immaturity and therefore reduced ability to excrete the breakdown products from excess red cells. The more preterm the infant, the earlier comes the point at which active treatment is required.

Respiratory assistance The preterm infant, with his immature lungs, is prone to respiratory difficulties, in particular respiratory distress syndrome or hyaline membrane disease. This is caused by low levels of surfactant, which is normally present to decrease surface tension in the alveoli, so allowing the lungs to fill with air. The baby with respiratory distress syndrome (RDS) grunts with his expiratory efforts and is tachypnoeic and cyanosed. His oxygen requirements are increased, but the amount given must be monitored carefully, since too much oxygen is as hazardous for the small baby as too little.

There are different means of providing respiratory assistance; all look very alarming to the new parents. The baby may have a nasal or oral endotracheal tube in position and be attached to a ventilator; he may receive some ventilatory support, with the use of intermittent mandatory ventilation (IMV); he may receive continuous positive airway pressure (CPAP) via the ventilator, via little plastic 'prongs' inserted into his nostrils, or by means of a face mask held in position with 'Netelast'.

The preterm or sick baby is prone to transient apnoea. Such a baby is nursed on an 'apnoea mattress'; this has an inbuilt device which sounds an alarm if the baby's chest movements cease.

Anaemia The preterm baby is prone to develop anaemia, because fetal iron stores increase during the last weeks of pregnancy. Preterm infants therefore receive iron and vitamin supplements.

The light-for-dates baby

The baby who is smaller than expected for the period of gestation may have had a poorly functioning placenta or he may be suffering from some abnormality. Placental insufficiency leads to poor nutrition and hypoxia, so that any further stresses may cause severe hypoxia and result in brain damage. Real efforts are made to monitor intrauterine growth, and the baby who appears to be suffering from intrauterine growth retardation needs to be delivered before such damage occurs. Many light-for-dates babies are very hungry after birth, demand frequent feeds, gain weight rapidly and have no further associated problems.

The light-for-dates baby does have a tendency to become hypoglycaemic. His liver will be small, and may not store sufficient glycogen for his metabolic needs.

HYPOGLYCAEMIA

Hypoglycaemia may occur in the light-for-dates baby, the baby of the diabetic mother, any baby whose first feed is delayed, or any baby who becomes chilled.

The baby of the diabetic mother has become accustomed to hyperglycaemia in his mother and therefore in him, prior to delivery. He therefore produces more insulin *in utero*, and will then become hypoglycaemic following delivery. The typical 'diabetic baby' is seen much less frequently today. It is now recognized that careful, maintained control of blood sugar during the pregnancy gives a much better outcome. The diabetic woman's baby used to be 'large for dates'—fat and lethargic. These were the babies who became hypoglycaemic very readily. Some women's diabetic control is very difficult to maintain during pregnancy, and so the problem does still exist.

The baby whose first feed is delayed or who becomes hypothermic depletes his glycogen stores in order to provide his energy needs.

Babies at risk of hypoglycaemia have their blood sugar estimated, using blood obtained from a heel prick, and 'Dextrostix' or 'BM stix'. This is repeated hourly or two-hourly if necessary, otherwise before feeds. Tube feeding may sometimes be necessary, and in severe hypoglycaemia, an intravenous infusion may be commenced. Feeds are offered at three- to four-hourly intervals, and demand feeding is not introduced until the risk period has passed, and the baby is alert and maintaining his blood sugar levels.

CONGENITAL ABNORMALITIES

Congenital malformations are numerous, though fortunately not extremely common, and a full list and description is outside the scope of this book. The reader is directed to more detailed textbooks of paediatrics if required.

Minor abnormalities

It is important to remember that a 'minor' abnormality may not seem at all minor to the parents, who had no thoughts other than producing a completely healthy baby.

Extra digits   These are sometimes seen. The extra digit usually contains little or no bone, and is ligated and separates without any problem.

Syndactyly   This is the term used to describe webbed or joined digits. It varies in severity and may need plastic surgery, but is often no shock, as it is usually prevalent in the family.

Birth marks   These vary in severity. Some fade and disappear, while others may require plastic surgery. Birthmarks may be a major handicap if they are extensive or disfiguring.

Major abnormalities

It is probably easiest to describe these system by system.

The skeletal system

Congenital dislocation of the hip   This is not necessarily a major problem, since early diagnosis dramatically
reduces the need for surgery. The hip test is performed
soon after birth, and then at least once more in the
early days. The examiner is looking for the typical
'click' of the hip which is unstable in the acetabulum.
It is more common in girls. The wearing of a splint
which maintains a position of abduction is necessary
for some weeks or months, and while this may seem
a minor matter to the doctor or nurse, the mother may
find it very awkward to manage this unwieldy baby,
who does not fit easily into the carry cot or baby chair,
and may be fretful and unsettled. Many of the clothes
she has bought may not be usable, and fitting nappies
may be difficult.

The limbs   Arms or legs may be malformed or absent.
The classic example was the phocomelia or amelia
caused by thalidomide prescribed to mothers in early
pregnancy in the 1960s.

Talipes (Fig. 18.1)   This may be a minor problem. The
baby who has had little room to move *in utero*, such as
one of a multiple pregnancy, or the baby surrounded
by very little liquor (oligohydramnios), may have a
positional talipes, where the feet are formed normally,
and are treated by physiotherapy alone. The more
severe forms involve developmental abnormalities of
the feet, and limitation of range of movement. Plaster
boots are normally fitted, but corrective surgery may
be necessary later in the first years of life.

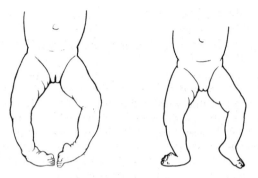

Fig. 18.1   Talipes equinovarus (left) and talipes calcaneovalgus (right).

The gastrointestinal tract

Cleft lip or palate   This too varies in severity (Fig. 18.2). In the worst cases the cleft is bilateral, so that there is a large defect in the hard palate, and the upper lip is very unsightly. The parents will be very shocked at delivery, but treatment is now excellent, and they may be reassured of this. A dental plate will be fitted within hours of birth, to provide some help with suck-

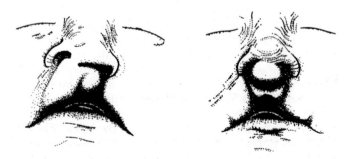

Fig. 18.2   Cleft lip: A, unilateral cleft lip; B, bilateral cleft lip.

ing. Without this, the baby will regurgitate his feed through his nose, a distressing experience for all. Plastic surgery is phased throughout the first years of life. Speech therapy may be needed later.

Tracheo-oesophageal fistula (TOF) This is suspected if the baby is very cyanosed and producing excessive mucus at birth. A nasogastric tube will not pass into the stomach. There are various manifestations; most commonly the oesophagus ends in a blind pouch. This condition requires major surgery within hours of birth, but these babies usually do very well.

Pyloric stenosis This does not manifest itself immediately, but is usually diagnosed at about six weeks. It is usually completely cured by Ramstedt's operation, where the pylorus is partially divided to relieve the stenosis.

Duodenal atresia The duodenum ends in a blind pouch. Surgical treatment is usually successful.

Imperforate anus This requires surgical treatment. If the sphincter is abnormal the child does not normally achieve good faecal continence, which is difficult for him and his family to live with.

Gastroschisis The stomach and gut protrude through the abdominal wall, which is incomplete. Surgery is performed as soon as possible.

Exomphalos This is a similar condition to gastroschisis; the gut herniates through a defect around the umbilicus.

The cardiovascular system

Cardiac anomalies are often multiple.

Ventricular septal defect (VSD)   This may not be diagnosed until a few weeks after birth.

Patent ductus arteriosus (PDA)   The ductus arteriosus is patent in the fetus, but closes within hours of birth; it may persist in the preterm baby.

Fallot's tetralogy   This consists of ventricular septal defect, pulmonary stenosis, overriding of the aorta and hypertrophy of the right ventricle.

Transposition of the great vessels   The positions of the pulmonary artery and the aorta are reversed. Treatment is surgical.

Coarctation of the aorta   The aorta narrows just after leaving the heart. Some cases are treated successfully by surgery.

The central nervous system

Hydrocephalus   This is often associated with spina bifida, but may occur alone. Its severity and prognosis varies tremendously, but in the less severe cases treatment may be very successful, though it may be ongoing.

Spina bifida   At present many doctors are not inclined to treat these babies actively if overall examination reveals a poor prognosis. The feelings of the parents must be taken into account.

The urogenital tract

Renal agenesis or Potter's syndrome   These babies may be born alive, but have other associated malformations, and do not survive more than a few hours.

Hypospadias   This is an abnormality of the penis, where the urethral meatus is on the ventral aspect of the penis, or even in the perineum. 'Chordee' is the term used to describe a curved penis.

Chromosomal abnormalities

Many fetuses with abnormal chromosomes abort spontaneously in early pregnancy.

Down's syndrome This is the commonest chromosomal abnormality, and occurs significantly more often in the baby of the older mother. The incidence rises sharply above a maternal age of 35 years. The baby has the typical mongoloid facies, with slanting eyes, wide epicanthus, protruding tongue, and is often 'floppy' and slow to feed. These children are always mentally retarded to some extent, but with intensive treatment many do extremely well. They usually have lovable, attractive personalities.

Other chromosomal abnormalities These include Turner's syndrome, where there is an abnormality of the sex chromosomes in girls; Patau's syndrome, and Edwards' syndrome.

Infection

Even a mild infection in the mother during the early weeks of pregnancy may have a devastating effect on embryonic development. Viruses such as rubella and cytomegalovirus may cause fetal abnormalities with brain damage.

BIRTH INJURIES

A difficult vaginal delivery (whether forceps or breech delivery) is avoided whenever possible in good obstetric practice, but sadly, birth injuries are still seen.

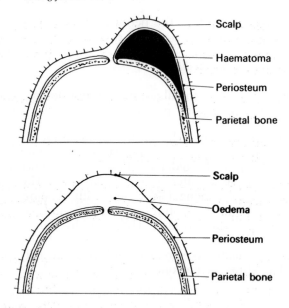

Fig. 18.3 Cross-section of a cephalhaematoma (above) and a caput succedaneum (below).

Bell's palsy This is a unilateral facial palsy, which subsides spontaneously.

Subdural haemorrhage This results from a tear in the cerebral membranes (the falx cerebri or the tentorium).

Cephalhaematoma This is a haematoma which forms between the periosteum and the underlying skull bone. It is differentiated from a 'caput succedaneum', which is seen on most babies after several hours of labour and is regarded as normal. The caput is surface tissue oedema, is present at birth and subsides within hours, or at most a couple of days; it may cross the suture lines. A cephalhaematoma, however, becomes noticeable within hours of the birth; it may then grow larger, it never crosses a suture line (though there may be bilateral cephalhaematomas) (Fig. 18.3). It may take some days to resolve.

Erb's palsy   This is a paralysis of one arm; recovery is usually complete.

Fractured clavicle   This may occur after difficulty delivering the shoulders (shoulder dystocia).

Forceps marks   These are present at birth following most forceps deliveries. They become more florid over the first hours of life, but will fade and disappear completely.

Bruising   The buttocks of a baby born by the breech may be bruised and oedematous, and following face presentation and delivery the face is also bruised and swollen. This looks very alarming, but parents may be reassured.

FURTHER READING

BRIMBLECOMBE, F. S. W., RICHARDS, M. P. M., & ROBERTON, N. R. C. (1978) *Separation and Special Care Baby Units*. London: Heinemann Medical Books.

CHISWICK, M. L. (1978) *Neonatal Medicine*, 1st edn. London: Update Publications.

HALLIDAY, H. L., McCLURE, G., & REID, M. (1985) *Handbook of Neonatal Intensive Care*, 2nd edn. London: Baillière Tindall.

KELNAR, C. J. H. & HARVEY, D. (1981) *The Sick Newborn Baby*. London: Baillière Tindall.

MOORE, K. L. (1983) *Before We Are Born* (Basic Embryology and Birth Defects). W. B. Saunders.

19

SOCIAL ASPECTS

STATISTICS AND DEFINITIONS

In order to understand the facts and figures relating to maternal and child health, it is important to know the definitions of various terms, and also to appreciate how such figures are compiled, particularly as not all are directly comparable.

Mortality rate   This is the death rate for a given population.

Morbidity rate   This is the disease or ill-health rate for a given population.

Infant mortality rate   This is the number of babies dying in the first year of life, per thousand *live* births.

Neonatal mortality rate   This is the number of babies dying in the first 28 days of life, per thousand *live* births.

Perinatal mortality rate   This is the number of babies dying in the first week of life, plus all stillbirths, per thousand *total* births.

Stillbirth rate   This is the number of babies born dead at or after 28 weeks' gestation, per thousand *total* births.

Maternal mortality rate   This is the number of women dying from causes associated with childbirth, per thousand *total* births.

The perinatal mortality rate is the statistic most often quoted when assessing the quality of health care offered to mothers and babies. Although perinatal mortality rates have fallen dramatically in the UK since the turn of the century, other countries in the West have been more successful in reducing these figures. One important factor in improving the perinatal mortality rate would be to improve antenatal care still further, to make it more personal, to give more care to those at risk, and to find ways of improving acceptance and uptake of care.

There are certain factors which increase the risk of perinatal mortality. These include: poor housing, low income, the unsupported parent, the very young mother, the older mother (usually quoted as over 35 years of age), the first pregnancy, high parity, and medical and obstetric complications.

HEALTH SERVICES AVAILABLE TO MOTHERS AND BABIES

One of the most important provisions made for pregnant women is the right to expert care before, during and after labour. Various recommendations since the early 1970s have stated that a hospital confinement is the safest and best for every woman. This is open to debate, and many consumers have voiced their dissatisfaction with both this assertion, and the provision itself. However, almost every woman in the UK does have her baby in hospital, even if she returns home almost immediately. Relatively few general practitioners will agree to give medical supervision to women wanting a home confinement, though the midwife has a statutory obligation to attend the woman in labour at home, even in the absence of medical support. This latter is not the ideal situation, of course, and every effort is usually made to find a compromise which offers safety to mother and baby, and is acceptable to the professionals and the couple. The options available to women are discussed in Chapter 7—'Antenatal care'.

The midwife

The midwife is specially trained and experienced in the care of women and their babies during normal pregnancy, labour, and the postnatal period. She (or he) is able to advise on a wide range of topics, and refers women to appropriate agencies if a matter is outside her scope. She is trained to detect abnormalities, and is expected to refer women promptly for medical advice or supervision when necessary.

In the past two decades midwives have had to adjust to a great many changes, in their training and their practice. Midwifery training involves an 18-month course, following registration as a general nurse at present. This length of time enables the student midwife to assimilate the varied, detailed knowledge which is essential to her safe practice.

There have also had to be deliberations on the needs of the midwife who may wish to work elsewhere within the EEC, and certain standards have been agreed within the member countries to give reciprocal recognition to all European midwives.

The supervising body at national level in the UK is the United Kingdom Central Council for nursing, midwifery and health visiting (the UKCC). Each country within the UK has its own Board, and each specialty has its own Committee on that Board. The UKCC issues 'Rules' and a 'Code of Practice' for midwives. At local authority level, there is a supervisor of midwives, who is responsible for the day-to-day super-vision and co-ordination of midwives in her area.

Like any other professional person, the midwife is accountable for her decisions and actions, and is liable to disciplinary procedures if there is any question arising from her practice.

Within each obstetric unit, policies are agreed between senior midwifery and obstetric staff, regarding details of the midwives' practice. Because obstetricians have become so prominent in the care of pregnant and labouring women since the early 1970s, the midwife has become somewhat undervalued, but she has a great deal to offer in the care of mothers and babies.

Benefits available during pregnancy

Financial benefits available to pregnant women re-mained unchanged for some years; until April 1987, every woman could obtain a Maternity Grant of £25, if she had been resident in the UK for the previous six months. From April 1987, this was revised, and a grant of £75 is now payable to women eligible on the grounds of need. The previously available 'special needs payment' will no longer be so readily obtainable.

Statutory Maternity Pay (SMP) is the main financial provision for working women. It is operated by the employer, in much the same way as Statutory Sick Pay. The woman must have been employed for a certain period of time, working sufficient hours, and earning enough to pay National Insurance contributions, in order to qualify for SMP. If a woman is not eligible for SMP, she is advised to claim Maternity Allowance.

Maternity Allowance is still payable to women who have been working, but who have recently changed jobs. The amount payable is dependent on the number of National Insurance stamps which she or her em-ployer had paid.

If a woman has worked for her employer for a period of two years, she is eligible for maternity leave, with her job being kept open for her. She should be able to leave work to attend the antenatal clinic without losing pay.

Free dental treatment and free prescriptions are available for the woman during her pregnancy, and until the baby is one year old.

Women receiving social security benefits can obtain free milk and vitamins.

Provisions available for mother and baby

The new mother and baby are discharged from hospital to the care of the primary health care team. This includes the general practitioner, the community midwife, the health visitor, and a wide range of other professionals, such as dentists, speech therapists, chiropodists, and the 'back up' staff essential to the smooth running of a surgery or health centre, such as the receptionists and secretaries.

The community midwife visits mother and baby at home until at least 10 days following delivery, though she may opt to visit until 28 days if she wishes, or if their condition warrants this. At the end of this time, she refers them to the care of the health visitor.

The health visitor is a registered nurse with particular training in preventive health care. She takes a special interest in the preschool child, though she is responsible for health care throughout the community, and may receive referrals of a widely varied nature.

She will visit mother and baby at home, but will also invite the mother to attend the baby clinic. She will monitor the baby's development, sometimes by performing formal tests, but also by observation, and questioning the mother. In some areas the doctor will perform all the formal developmental checks. The health visitor is able to refer mother and baby for specialist help and advice when necessary.

At the baby clinic, the mother may have her baby weighed; she may see the health visitor if she wishes, and in most clinics she may have the baby immunized at the appropriate times. Some general practitioners will prefer to follow up children in their practice themselves. If this is not so, developmental assessments are carried out by the doctor at the clinic, who is employed for the purpose by the local health authority. General medical problems are referred to the general practitioner at his surgery.

In many areas the health visitor is 'attached' to a particular general practice, and this enables close, effective liaison in many cases. On the other hand, the health visitor may cover a geographical area, and this enables her to get to know all the mothers in the neighbourhood well, and to become a trusted, well used professional if she takes the time to build up trusting relationships.

Child care

For the woman who needs or wishes to return to work, or who finds it difficult to cope with her family, there is a certain amount of help available.

Child minder   This is an informal provision, where a woman, often with small children herself, cares for children during the day. She should be registered with the Social Services Department, who will inspect her home, and will place a limit on the number of children who may be cared for at any one time. In some areas there is a provision known as 'sponsored child minding' where child minding costs are subsidized by the local authority for families with special needs, such as those at risk of child abuse.

Mother and toddler group   This is an informal provision, where mothers can meet over tea or coffee, and toddlers can run around and play.

Playgroup   This is another informal provision. Children are admitted from the age of about three years, and are given opportunity to play with other small children, as well as having some group activities, such as organized games, stories and singing. This gives a social outlet for both mother and child. An 'opportunity playgroup' is one which caters for handicapped children, usually admitting normal children as well.

Day nursery or Nursery Centres   This is a provision for which the Social Services Department is responsible. Places tend to be limited, and many are allocated to children at risk of child abuse or to those with other 'special needs' such as mental handicap. Ideally the nursery staff should aim to work with the parents as well as the child or children.

Nursery school   This provision is not a statutory one; it is run by the education services, and its availability varies across the country.

Foster care   At times of crisis families may need outside help, and foster care is a means of providing this. Foster parents are vetted by the Social Services Department, and receive some financial help from them. Foster care is provided for the baby who is to be adopted.

Child abuse

Child abuse is an age-old problem, which receives much more publicity at the present time. Abuse may be physical or emotional, and sexual abuse is a problem which is receiving much more attention now.

Professionals should always be alert to the possibility of child abuse, or the family at risk, i.e. the family under stress, but the 'label' should be used with the utmost care.

Each local authority lays down its own guidelines and procedures for dealing with suspected or potential child abuse. Referrals may come from any individual, lay or professional. The National Society for the Prevention of Cruelty to Children (the NSPCC) has an important role in caring for families at risk, and they deal with many such referrals.

Screening

'Screening' is the scrutiny of a particular population, looking for a specific disease. The screening programme must be efficient and cost-effective. The disease must be easy to diagnose, and must be treatable once detected. In political terms this includes facilities and finance. Examples of routine screening programmes for babies include the following.

The Guthrie test   Every baby is tested for phenylketonuria at the age of seven days (or in the case of the sick or preterm baby, when he has been receiving milk feeds for seven days). Blood is placed on a special card, from a heel prick, and tested in the laboratory.

The hip test   This is to detect congenital dislocation of the hip, and is performed at least once in the neonatal period, and usually repeated at three months of age.

The hearing test   The health visitor normally performs this on every baby at about seven months of age.

Mothers also receive screening tests in the antenatal period, and after the baby is born. For many women their first pregnancy provides the first contact they have had with medical and preventive services for many years. For women who have attended the Family Planning Clinic, cervical smears and blood pressure checks have become routine. If a woman has not had a cervical smear performed, the antenatal booking clinic gives an opportunity for this test to be performed.

The various blood tests which are performed also provide a screening programme for this particular population, and include testing for rubella antibodies, Rhesus factor and increasingly, for such antibodies as hepatitis B and HIV. It should be noted, however, that routine screening for HIV is not carried out in the UK. Although there has been discussion about anonymously examining excess blood from routine sampling in order to assess the prevalence of HIV-positive individuals in the country, nurses and midwives have received strongly worded guidelines stating that any such testing should only be carried out with the individual's *informed* consent.

'Well woman clinics' are available in most areas, some run privately. These provide a cervical smear service and general health checks. Women should also be taught self-examination of the breasts, and be encouraged to carry this out monthly.

FURTHER READING

Babies and Benefits. DHSS leaflet FB8.
BENNETT, V. R. & BROWN, L. K. (Eds.) (1989) *Myles Textbook for Midwives*, 11th edn. Edinburgh: Churchill Livingstone.
CLARK, J. & HENDERSON, J. (1989) *Community Health*. Edinburgh: Churchill Livingstone.
HOUSTON, M. J. (Ed.) (1984) *Maternal and Infant Health Care* (Recent Advances in Nursing—9). Edinburgh: Churchill Livingstone.
MEREDITH-DAVIES, J. B. (1975) *Community Health, Preventive Medicine and Social Services*, 3rd edn. London: Baillière Tindall.
ORR, J. (Ed.) (1987) *Women's Health in the Community* (Topics in Community Health). Chichester: John Wiley.

Gynaecology

20

GYNAECOLOGICAL EXAMINATION AND INVESTIGATIONS

ASSESSMENT

Assessment of a patient with a disorder of the reproductive system includes taking a history and a physical examination.

History

Information is obtained about the following:

1. History of any disorders, illnesses, injuries, surgery and diagnostic investigations of the reproductive system.
2. History and character of menstruation (including: menarche, last menstrual period, length of cycle, duration of flow, amount of flow, menopause and last cervical smear test).
3. History of reproductive events [including: number of pregnancies and the outcome of these (abortion, preterm, full-term), delivery (types), children (any still-birth or neonatal death and cause if known), present health status, complications of pregnancy, history of infertility and cause if known, and present and past use of contraception)].
4. Review of function. In reviewing a system questioning should elicit:

(a) Any changes or disturbances in function (for example, dysmenorrhoea, dissatisfaction with sexual functioning or birth control).
(b) The presence of any symptoms of disease. If symptoms are present they are explored in order to determine their location, character, duration and severity. The common manifestations of disorders are: pain, lesions, discharges, itching, non-cyclic bleeding, swellings and masses.

Physical examination

The physical examination includes:

1. General physical examination.
2. Inspection of secondary sexual characteristics see Fig. 20.1.
3. Inspection and palpation of internal and external genitalia see Fig. 20.2

The vaginal examination is often a source of anxiety for women. The examination is personal and invades body boundaries and there is a sense of exposure. For these reasons the individual having her first vaginal examination should be prepared in advance for what is involved. The examination procedure is described and she is shown the equipment. The patient undergoing a vaginal examination may have a sense of physical and emotional exposure; the nurse can help to reduce these feelings by her sensitive and supportive approach.

IDENTIFICATION OF PATIENT PROBLEMS

The patient with a disorder of the reproductive system presents some special concerns for the nurse. In many ways a human being is defined by his sex. Knowing he

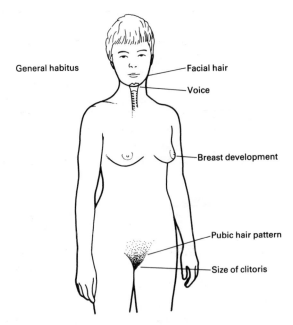

Fig. 20.1 Inspection of secondary sex characteristics forms part of this examination. (A deep voice, facial trichosis, hypoplastic breasts, a tendency to male escutcheon, and an enlarged clitoris suggest the need for studies to exclude a masculinizing lesion of the pituitary, adrenals, or ovaries.)

or she is a man or a woman gives the person a set of behaviours, culturally and physiologically determined, which help to guide his or her actions. The normal functioning of the reproductive system gives constant reassurance of a person's essential maleness or femaleness. The distortion or interruption of these processes may prove very disturbing to the individual and family.

The person may experience problems in relation to his or her self-image and have fears about future sexual performance and attractiveness. Body parts that con-

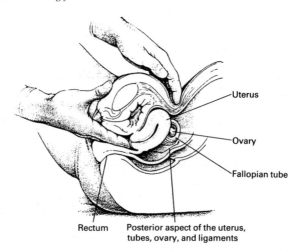

Uterus

Ovary

Fallopian tube

Rectum   Posterior aspect of the uterus,
tubes, ovary, and ligaments

Fig. 20.2   Bimanual vaginal examination.

tribute to self-esteem and identity have a high psychological investment. The threat posed by loss of these body parts depends on:

1. Their meaning to the individual.
2. His or her stage of development of body image and self.
3. The reactions of the social group to which he or she belongs, including the sexual partner.

The person may fear loss of reproductive function. The ability to reproduce is seen by many as a criterion of usefulness and sexuality. The loss of function may be followed by feelings of uselessness or of being only half a person. These feelings can be particularly distressing to the woman who has defined herself in terms of her reproductive and sexual function. To her the removal of her uterus or ovaries may be tantamount to removing her femaleness. Because she may feel less a woman, she fears her partner will see her as less a woman. Indeed, in some unfortunate situations, they may. Thus, to the fear of loss of reproductive function may be added the fear of loss of a loved one. For some the fear of loss of libido as well as sexual function may be very frightening and can cause the patient much anguish.

Also, most patients have been culturally conditioned to the idea that these areas of the body should not be discussed, much less exposed, in examination or discussion. Such experiences may disturb the individual and produce shame that may be enhanced by lack of privacy and exposure of the body in examinations or during care. Other patients may feel guilt over their illness. Venereal disease, abortion and cancer arouse guilt feelings in certain individuals which may be expressed as a feeling of 'being punished for past deeds'.

The nurse deals with patients who experience anxiety and fear, shame, guilt, diminished self-esteem or re-awakened anxieties over personal identity.

When caring for such patients the *goals* are to:

1. Promote feelings of self-worth at both the personal and sexual level.
2. Assist the individual to a resolution of dys-functional sexual problems.
3. Avoid practices that contribute to shame.
4. Relieve guilt.
5. Help the individual overcome body image disturbances.
6. Increase the patient's knowledge of relevant anatomy and physiology.
7. Dispel misconceptions.

Nursing intervention

These goals may be achieved by the following nursing interventions. The nurse should:

1. Assess the degree of threat posed by loss of function or body parts to the individual and plan, give and evaluate nursing care for that individual based on the assessment.
2. Give physical nursing care which:
(a) Promotes feelings of dignity, self-worth and attractiveness by attention to personal hygiene and grooming.
(b) Promotes the return of health, control over body functions and independence.
3. Reduce fear and guilt by:
(a) Acknowledging and discussing feelings.
(b) Anticipating the need for explanations and interpretations.
(c) Clarifying and correcting misinformation about causes of illness, physiology and the consequences, if any, of treatment on present function.
(d) Maintaining a confident, non-judgemental approach to the patient.
(e) Assisting in acknowledging the loss, if any.
(f) Obtaining appropriate additional sources of spiritual or emotional help for the patient.

EXPECTED OUTCOMES

Interventions are successful if behavioural changes have occurred, although behavioural changes may be difficult to document in areas such as self-concept, anxiety and guilt. The patient:

1. States that she feels better, less frightened or happier.

2. Takes an interest in her appearance and renews interests in her social life, which may also indicate a return to a more positive outlook toward the future.

3. Demonstrates an understanding of her illness, treatments and any residual changes in function to the level of her ability or willingness.

4. Demonstrates a knowledge of the risk factors which may lead to a recurrence of the problem and the actions which may reduce or eliminate the risk factors, if appropriate.

5. Discusses her altered body with the nurse and so indicates a willingness to begin to deal with the problem or to accept it with appropriate adjustments.

Adjustment to many of these changes requires some time and complete resolution is rarely seen in hospital. Expectations of resolution and effectiveness of intervention must be realistic.

In all this the nurse should endeavour to avoid repetition of the doctor's examination and history taking or the woman will begin to feel she is under interrogation.

The nurse will also be responsible for assisting the doctor as he examines the patient, both in the ward and the out-patient clinic. She will need to become familiar with some of the special positions and instruments used.

The doctor will usually perform a bimanual examination. Here he is using both hands to palpate internally and externally to elicit masses or tenderness.

POSITIONS

Dorsal The patient lies on her back with her head supported on one pillow, the knees flexed and apart (Fig. 20.3). This position is the one most commonly

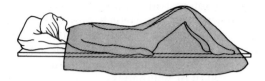

Fig. 20.3   Dorsal position.

used for abdominal, vulval, vaginal and bimanual examinations.

Left lateral   The patient lies on her left side with the buttocks on the edge of the bed, her knees bent with the right knee drawn up higher than the left, and her head supported on one pillow (Fig. 20.4). This position may be used for vaginal, vulval and rectal examinations, taking vaginal swabs or cervical smears, or for a normal delivery.

Sims' position   This is an exaggerated left lateral position where the left arm is placed behind the back and the right knee is drawn up further (Fig. 20.5). This tilts the pelvis and trunk further so giving easier access for inserting a vaginal pack or pessary. The left arm should be positioned with care or the patient may later suffer from pain in the shoulder.

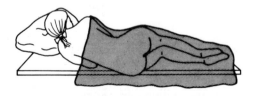

Fig. 20.4   Left lateral position.

Lithotomy position   The patient lies on her back with the legs abducted, the heels supported in stirrups on poles at the side of the bed or table (Fig. 20.6). Once the patient is positioned the lower end of the table is removed and the buttocks brought to the edge of the table. This position is used for operations on the vagina, vulva or rectum, and for forceps delivery. The patient may have been given a regional or general anaesthetic and her legs must be positioned with care.

Special points:

Socks should be worn to protect the ankles.
Both legs must be flexed simultaneously onto the abdomen and then the feet placed outside the poles and into the stirrups.

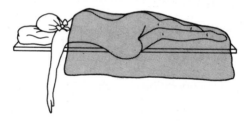

Fig. 20.5   Sims' position.

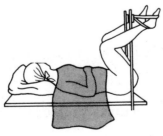

Fig. 20.6   Lithotomy position.

If the legs are moved separately sacro-iliac strain may be caused.

The calves should be positioned so that they are not pressed against the poles, or venous return may be impeded.

The hips should not be abducted beyond the point of resistance, particularly in the older woman. Great care should be taken if the patient has arthritis, or back or hip problems.

Genupectoral or knee–chest position The patient kneels on the bed, bends forward and rests her head and shoulders on a pillow so that her thighs are vertical to the bed and the pelvis is as high as possible (Fig. 20.7).

The main use for this position is to relieve pressure on a prolapsed cord in obstetrics.

Trendelenburg position The patient is recumbent on the table which is then tilted head downwards (Fig. 20.8). This displaces the abdominal contents against the diaphragm allowing easier access to the pelvic organs for operations such as caesarean section, hysterectomy and oophorectomy.

EQUIPMENT USED FOR EXAMINATION

The following are required for vaginal examination:

 a length of paper towel which is placed under the
    buttocks
 disposable gloves
 antiseptic lotion
 lubricants—Hibitane cream and KY jelly
 a selection of specula—*Sims'*, *Cusco's*, and *Fergusson's*
    in various sizes

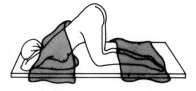

Fig. 20.7   Genupectoral position.

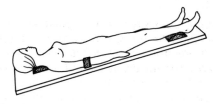

Fig. 20.8   Trendelenburg position.

  cotton wool balls
  sponge-holders
  receptacle or bag for used instruments
  disposable bag for used gloves and swabs

Vaginal examination is normally a sterile procedure if the patient is aborting, in labour, postpartum or postoperatively.

In addition the following are required for obtaining vaginal or cervical specimens:

  sterile culture swabs
  Stuart's transport medium
  Ayre spatula (or similar)
  microscope slides with frosted glass end
  a lead pencil
  special fixative solution
  transport boxes
  pathology and histology request forms

An anglepoise lamp is also required.

A high vaginal swab is taken if infection is present or suspected.

A cervical smear may be taken during the examination if the patient has not had one taken within the previous three to five years and is sexually active. It is a test for early detection of carcinoma of the cervix, which responds well to treatment in the early stages. The cervical canal is lined with columnar epithelium, while the cervical os is covered with a layer of stratified squamous epithelium. The two types of cells meet at the squamocolumnar junction, and when taking a cervical smear the aim is to obtain a sample of both types. Early precancerous changes may be detected on histological examination and surveillance of the patient and early treatment are vital in preventing the progress of the disease.

The special glass slide is labelled clearly with the patient's name, date of birth and hospital number,

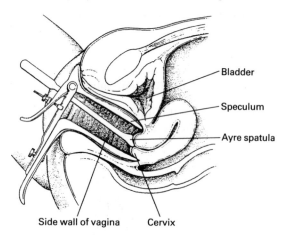

Fig. 20.9   Internal vaginal examination demonstrating the position of the speculum and Ayre spatula used to obtain cervical cells for a smear test.

using the lead pencil on the frosted end. Once the cervix is clearly visualized the Ayre spatula is inserted gently into the cervical os and rotated through 360° (Fig. 20.9). An alternative to the spatula is a specially designed small brush. The sample of cells is spread thinly and evenly on the glass slide, fixative is applied and allowed to dry before the slide is placed in a transport box.

SOME GYNAECOLOGICAL INSTRUMENTS

Cusco's speculum (Fig. 20.10) is used to expose the cervix for inspection or to take samples such as cervical secretions. The speculum is lubricated and inserted in the closed position into the vagina, rotated and then opened to separate the anterior and posterior vaginal walls. The patient is in the dorsal position.

Sims' speculum (Fig. 20.11) is used to retract the posterior vaginal wall and expose the cervix, for example when packing or painting the vagina. The end should be lubricated and passed along the posterior vaginal wall. The patient is in the left lateral position.

Ayre spatula (Fig. 20.12) is used to take a Papanicolaou's smear; the reverse end may be used to obtain a specimen from the vaginal fornices. It is a wooden or

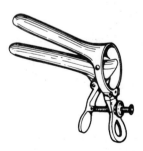

Fig. 20.10   Cusco's speculum.

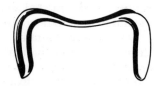

Fig. 20.11   Sims' speculum.

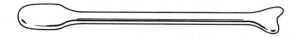

Fig. 20.12   Ayre spatula.

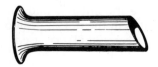

Fig. 20.13   Fergusson's speculum.

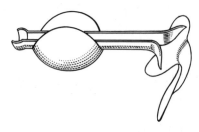

Fig. 20.14   Auvard's speculum.

plastic spatula, so designed that the longer portion is passed into the cervical canal and rotated. This collects cells from the squamocolumnar junction, the point where carcinoma is most likely to commence.

Fergusson's speculum (Fig. 20.13) is used when more support is required than can be given by the bivalve speculum. It is essentially just a metal tube which supports prolapsed vaginal walls to allow a view of the cervix. The patient is in the left lateral position.

Auvard's speculum (Fig. 20.14) is a weighted vaginal retractor and is only used in the operating theatre when the patient is anaesthetized.

Vulsellum forceps (Fig. 20.15) have large teeth which can grasp the cervix and allow traction to be exerted during procedures requiring the passage of an instrument through the cervical canal.

Hegar's dilators (Fig. 20.16) may be single or double ended and consist of a set of progressive sizes (1 to 16). They are passed through the cervical canal in turn in order to dilate it.

Uterine curettes (Figs. 20.17 and 20.18) may have a sharp or blunt end, may be double ended or flushing. These are passed into the uterus in order to scrape a specimen from the lining. The flushing curette allows for irrigation at the same time.

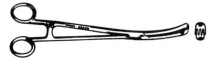

Fig. 20.15   Vulsellum forceps.

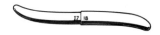

Fig. 20.16   Hegar's dilator.

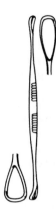

Fig. 20.17   Uterine curette.

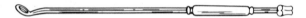

Fig. 20.18   Flushing curette.

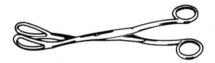

Fig. 20.19   Ovum forceps.

Ovum forceps (Fig. 20.19) are shaped like two spoons, which grasp the abortus or other debris and aid its removal from the uterine cavity.

Uterine sound (Fig. 20.20) is a long, thin instrument with graduations. This is passed into the uterus in order to measure its length.

Female bladder sound (Fig. 20.21) has no graduations and is fatter and shorter than a male bladder sound. It is used to estimate the size of the bladder.

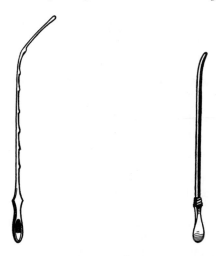

Fig. 20.20   Uterine sound   Fig. 20.21   Female bladder sound.

CONCLUSION OF EXAMINATION

When the doctor has finished his examination the patient should be given the opportunity to dress and regain her composure before he discusses his findings with her. At the very least she should be covered and encouraged to make herself comfortable. She will feel less at a disadvantage psychologically if she sits up. The nurse may need to facilitate discussion by encouraging the patient to ask questions, by interpreting the doctor's terminology if inappropriate or by asking the doctor to explain himself more clearly or in more detail if necessary.

The nurse may need to arrange for the doctor to see the patient's partner or family. Admission to hospital for further investigations, surgery or treatment may pose difficulties for the mother with young children, and the nurse may need to enlist the help of the hospital social worker.

PSYCHOLOGICAL PREPARATION FOR SURGERY

Research has shown that giving women information about forthcoming surgery helps them cope with the anticipation and the surgery itself much better. They need to know what to expect in terms of preoperative preparation and postoperative events, both in the short and the longer term. Suggesting ways they may help themselves is positive.

Reactions to change in body image and self-esteem have been discussed earlier in this chapter and the woman needs to be prepared for these.

FURTHER INVESTIGATIONS

Ultrasound scanning   This is a very important diagnostic aid in both obstetrics and gynaecology. High frequency sound waves directed at a particular organ or group of organs will bounce off different types of tissue in different ways. The resulting pattern can be 'translated' into a picture on a screen. In order to push the pelvic organs slightly out of the pelvis so that they may be visualized the woman must arrive in the ultrasound department with a full bladder. Uses of ultrasound include confirmation of ovulation and of pregnancy, dating of pregnancy, monitoring of fetal growth; diagnosis of multiple pregnancy, hydatidiform mole, abnormalities or neoplasms of the genital tract, pelvic abscess, retained products of conception.

Dilatation and curettage (D & C)   This is the most commonly performed gynaecological operation. With the patient anaesthetized and in the lithotomy position the cervix is dilated using progressively larger dilators, and the endometrium is scraped or aspirated. This may be therapeutic or diagnostic. D & C may be performed in the investigation of infertility, abnormal uterine bleeding or to remove retained products of conception.

Endometrial biopsy This may be performed using a special instrument. Dilatation of the cervix is not necessary and so it is a quick, simple diagnostic procedure.

VABRA aspiration sampling This is a new technique used to obtain a sample of endometrium for biopsy.

Laparoscopy This is another very important advance in gynaecology since it has reduced the incidence of laparotomy in diagnosis. It is performed in the operating theatre under general anaesthetic. The table is tilted so that the patient is in the Trendelenburg position. A trocar is introduced through a small sub-umbilical incision and carbon dioxide is blown into the abdomen to displace the gut and give a clear view of the pelvic organs. A uterine sound is often passed into the uterus, or vulsellum forceps are attached to the cervix to allow manipulation of the uterus by an assistant. The laparoscope has a fibreoptic light source and the operator can visualize the pelvic organs. Certain procedures may be carried out via the laparoscope. These include clipping of the fallopian tubes (female sterilization), removal of oocytes for *in vitro* fertilization (IVF), replacement of the fertilized ovum in gamete intrafallopian transfer (GIFT) and diathermy of endometriosis.

The carbon dioxide is absorbed into the tissues and excreted fairly rapidly, but may be the cause of some postoperative discomfort.

Colposcopy   This procedure permits magnified visualization of vaginal and cervical tissue. It may be performed in the out-patient department. The vagina and cervix may be stained with different substances so that abnormal cells show, and areas for biopsy are delineated. Patients with early precancerous changes on cervical smear will be examined by this means.

Cervitography   A special camera is used via the colposcope to photograph any suspicious areas of the cervix. In some centres nurses are trained to perform this procedure.

Hysteroscopy   Visual examination of the uterine cavity facilitates investigation of pelvic pain, infertility, abnormal uterine bleeding and neoplasms of the uterus.

Culdoscopy   This method of visualizing pelvic organs via the pouch of Douglas by passing a culdoscope through the posterior fornix of the vagina has been largely superseded by laparoscopy, which is much more versatile.

FURTHER READING

GOULD, D. (1990) *Nursing Care of Women*. Englewood Cliffs, NJ: Prentice-Hall.

GOVAN, A. D. *et al.* (1985) *Gynaecology Illustrated*. 3rd edn. Edinburgh: Churchill Livingstone.

SIMONS, W. (1985) *Learning to Care on the Gynaecology Ward*. Sevenoaks: Hodder & Stoughton.

WATSON, J. E. & ROYLE, J. R. (1987) *Watson's Medical-Surgical Nursing, and Related Physiology*, 3rd edn. London: Bailliére Tindall.

WEBB, C. (Ed.) (1986) *Women's Health. Midwifery and Gynaecological Nursing* (Using Nursing Models Series). Sevenoaks: Hodder & Stoughton.

WEBB, C. & WILSON-BARNETT, J. (1983) Hysterectomy: a study in coping with recovery. *Journal of Advanced Nursing*, **8**, 311–319.

21

PRE- AND POSTOPERATIVE CARE

The detailed preparation and after-care of women for any surgical procedure will vary from one centre to another, and will vary within individual units depending on the preferences of individual gynaecologists.

It is important to remember that women about to undergo the same gynaecological procedure may have very different needs, and so within the framework of unit policies there should be room for individualized care.

This is met to some extent by the use of the nursing process, but even this attempt at providing care to meet each patient's particular needs lends itself to automation and repetition. Planning care to suit each woman takes time and effort, but if well done will make the woman's experience of hospital life more personalised and less traumatic. Nurses generally still have to make an effort to move away from task allocation to seeing the whole patient and her needs if they are to achieve these ideals. Most units devise some form of care plan for use with gynaecological patients. Two very useful 'models' are those described by Orem and by Roper, Tierney and Logan.

The Orem model is based on self-care, and aims to enable the patient to care for herself as much as possible as soon as possible. This means of planning care also embraces the concept of individuals taking responsibility for their own health care, and making decisions where appropriate.

The model devised by Roper, Tierney and Logan is based on the activities of daily living, aiming to assess how far the patient is able to carry these out, and to find ways to assist her in resuming these progressively and realistically.

Nursing care should be based on research findings rather than tradition. Many practices have recently been shown to be less than useful but are still carried out faithfully in hospital wards. Examples include the use of salt baths, preoperative shaving in some instances and certain aspects of wound care.

Some practices are valid in themselves but are carried out without due thought and attention. An example of this is preoperative starving of patients. This is a necessary measure, but only for four hours pre-operatively. It is common for all patients to be deprived of food and drink from midnight prior to the next morning's surgical list, despite the fact that not all the patients can be operated on concurrently. This means that the first patient is starved for at least eight hours, and the last patient on the list may be starved for up to 12 or 13 hours, when she could have had a light breakfast. This is not to say that the first patient should be woken at 4 a.m. for a snack, but she could have tea and biscuits if she is unable to sleep, for example. The unfortunate patient who is last on the list is probably most likely to have her operation cancelled if an emergency arises, and she may then have to suffer similarly on the following day. Individualized care would include giving a light meal at the appropriate time in order to maintain hydration and blood sugar levels.

Gynaecological operations can be considered under the headings of major abdominal surgery, minor abdominal surgery, vaginal surgery, and various minor procedures.

PREOPERATIVE CARE

Preparation for major abdominal surgery

Major abdominal surgery includes abdominal hysterectomy with or without salpingo-oophorectomy, myomectomy, diagnostic laparotomy, pelvic exenteration, oophorectomy or ovarian cystectomy and tubal surgery aimed at restoring tubal patency.

Vulval shaving A pubic shave is necessary for a Pfannenstiel incision, but research has shown that the incidence of postoperative infection is increased by the presence of tiny nicks in the skin after shaving. Shaving must therefore be carried out with care, and the area shaved must be no more extensive than is required for adequate skin cleansing and surgical access in the operating theatre. The old 'through shave' is not necessary; once an adequate area has been shaved, remaining hair may be clipped if desirable. Shaving also adds to postoperative discomfort as the hair grows again. There may be a place for depilatory creams, though skin sensitivity will be a problem for some patients.

Bowel preparation Although some surgeons may prefer every patient to receive some form of bowel preparation it is much better to give this according to individual needs. The woman who is constipated will need suppositories during the evening before operation; if the patient can empty her bowels naturally beforehand she does not need artificial help which will cause her unnecessary discomfort.

Urinary catheterization This is usually carried out in the operating theatre.

Preoperative starving The patient should be asked not to eat or drink for four hours prior to induction of anaesthesia. A clear explanation of the reasons will result in greater compliance.

Vaginal douching This is considered out-moded in the UK and is rarely if ever performed as a preoperative measure.

Hygiene The woman is asked to have a bath about two hours before the expected time of operation. She is given a clean gown to wear.

Premedication This is given as prescribed by the anaesthetist, usually in cooperation with operating theatre staff, who will advise ward staff of progress and anticipated timing of operations.

Jewellery and make-up The woman is asked to remove these. Any valuables should ideally be taken home, but if the woman has them with her they should be locked away safely, duly labelled and documented. Some women will be unable or unwilling to remove jewellery such as gold bangles, and these and wedding rings are covered with adhesive tape. Theatre staff are responsible for ensuring that no metal object on the patient is touched by diathermy.

Preparation for minor abdominal surgery

Minor abdominal surgery includes abdominal tubal ligation and laparoscopy. Preparation for these procedures is as described in the preceding paragraph, bearing in mind individual needs.

Preparation for vaginal surgery

Vaginal surgery includes vaginal hysterectomy, any kind of pelvic floor repair and any combination of the two. Vulvectomy is not strictly vaginal surgery, but will be considered in this section.

Bowel preparation   An empty bowel is necessary for these procedures and for the woman's well-being in the postoperative period.

Pubic shaving   Clipping of the pubic and vulval hair is probably adequate, except for vulvectomy, when a complete shave will be required.

Other preoperative measures will be as already described in the preceding paragraphs.

Preparation for minor procedures

Minor procedures include dilatation and curettage (D & C), colposcopy, laser treatment, cryosurgery, avulsion of polyps, termination of pregnancy, marsupialization of Bartholin's cyst, endometrial biopsy, biopsy of the cervix, cervical cerclage (Shirodkar suture).

Many of these procedures will be carried out on an out-patient basis and the woman will be able to go home on the same day. Some patients will require an overnight stay. Preoperative preparation will be minimal and a full care plan is not necessary though individual care should still be the aim.

Other aspects of preoperative care

Other aspects of preoperative care include the contribution of the physiotherapist, any medical investigations such as blood tests and chest X-rays and the preoperative assessment by the anaesthetist.

Psychological preparation

Any period spent in hospital will be stressful for the individual concerned, and any means available to reduce that stress will be much appreciated. The giving of information is a well-recognized and obvious means of reducing stress, and every patient should be given as full an explanation of her condition, the planned treatment and the expected outcome as is possible.

Some women will want less information; this wish should be respected, and the assurance given that the opportunity is there for her to ask further details if she wishes.

It is important for a woman to have the opportunity to discuss the long-term effects of her condition and its treatment. Gynaecological surgery has important implications for a woman's self-image, her sexuality and therefore her self-confidence. She may have serious worries as to her future sexual activity, her attractiveness, and her ability to maintain an existing or future relationship. She will need time, privacy, the certainty of confidentiality and a sympathetic ear in order to voice such concerns.

POSTOPERATIVE CARE

As with preoperative care, postoperative care must be given according to the individual's needs, and not under a 'blanket' policy. Once again this involves seeing the woman as a whole individual and assessing her requirements.

Baseline observations Temperature, pulse, blood pressure, respiratory rate and colour should be recorded on the patient's return from the recovery room. More specialized monitoring may include reading a central venous pressure line. The anaesthetist may have given specific instructions for the immediate recovery period and these must be carried out intelligently. He should be notified of any significant change in the patient's condition.

Observation of the wound   The wound should be inspected at appropriate intervals, though removing the dressing is not necessary. If the dressing becomes soaked with exudate or blood it should be covered with a further absorbent sterile dressing and the doctor informed. All drains should be checked.

Vaginal loss   The vulval pad should be inspected at the same time as all other observations, and the nature and volume of the loss noted. Apparently excessive loss should be assessed by a skilled eye, and the doctor informed. A vaginal pack may be inserted in theatre at the end of some vaginal procedures and any drainage seeping through the pack should be noted. When the vaginal pack is removed, usually after 24 hours, vaginal loss must be observed as there is a risk of bleeding.

Urinary catheter   This may be a urethral or suprapubic catheter. Catheter toilet will be carried out by careful washing around the urethral orifice. There is less risk of ascending infection with a suprapubic catheter. Another advantage is that residual urine may be measured by clamping the catheter and asking the woman to pass urine, whereas the procedure with a urethral catheter involves removing the catheter and inserting a new one if the patient cannot empty her bladder adequately. A fluid balance chart is maintained and any apparent failure of the catheter to drain is noted and reported. Any haematuria is reported to the doctor.

Analgesia   The nurse is the best person to assess the adequacy or otherwise of postoperative pain relief. It should be possible for every patient to receive sufficient analgesia, and this should be given with thought. A different prescription should be sought if necessary. Analgesia may be combined with an anti-emetic.

Fluid balance   An intravenous infusion will be in progress after major abdominal surgery and oral fluids are recommenced when bowel sounds are heard. Some patients will have a blood transfusion in progress.

Diet   A light diet is offered once bowel sounds are heard after major surgery.

Bowel care   A stool softener may be required to initiate and maintain normal bowel action. Constipation and straining at stool should be avoided, since this will be traumatic as well as unpleasant for the woman.

Ambulation   Major surgery carries the risk of deep vein thrombosis and its sequelae, particularly for the older woman, and early ambulation is desirable. The woman should be helped to the toilet and bathroom as soon as she feels able.

Hygiene   Women will prefer to care for their own hygiene needs as soon as possible. The use of the bidet should be explained where appropriate. A detachable shower head is an alternative means of self-care for vulval toilet. Vulval hygiene for the woman still in bed may be given using a jug to pour water over the vulva while she lies on a bed-pan and then drying the area gently with sterile Gamgee or gauze. Alternatively, the vulval area may simply be washed and dried. A sterile vulval pad is then left in place.

Special points

Although the woman may feel 'less of a woman' after a hysterectomy, tubal ligation or other gynaecological surgery, the most obviously mutilating operation is vulvectomy. An important aspect of care here is to prepare the woman for seeing her wound for the first time. Both she and her partner will feel very apprehensive about this and she should not be forced to look at the operation site until she feels ready.

Vulvectomy wounds are often slow to heal. The patient is usually an older woman, and mobilization is important, though not always easy. The wound may drain copiously, there is usually at least one vacuum drain in place, and the urinary catheter will remain in place for up to two weeks.

Advice on discharge

Women need practical, succinct advice on discharge from hospital. Rather than a vague 'no lifting' directive, they need to be told exactly how long they should ask someone else to do the weekly shopping. Advice should be given on good lifting techniques generally.

'Light' housework such as dusting without stretching or bending is acceptable activity on discharge, and the woman must not be encouraged to assume the invalid role. She should be encouraged to resume normal activity gradually. The problem for many women is the dependent family who will not offer support and help, but who see the wife and mother as the indispensable linchpin of the home. In this case the family need firm guidance, and perhaps some outside assistance, such as a home help, for a time.

Every woman should be advised to take an afternoon rest with her feet up for a few weeks after major gynaecological surgery. She is normally advised not to have sexual intercourse until after her out-patient appointment about six weeks post-operatively. She is similarly advised not to drive a car.

She should be advised of the possible emotional sequelae, mood swings, tearfulness or depression, and she may appreciate the address of an appropriate support group.

She should also be alerted to the signs and symptoms of possible complications such as urinary tract infection or secondary haemorrhage, and advised when to seek medical help.

FURTHER READING

SIMONS, W. (1985) *Learning to Care on the Gynaecology Ward.* Sevenoaks: Hodder & Stoughton.

WATSON, J. E. & ROYLE, J. R. (Eds.) (1987) *Watson Medical-Surgical Nursing and Related Physiology*, 3rd edn. London: Baillière Tindall.

WEBB, C. (1986) *Women's Health. Midwifery and Gynaecological Nursing* (Using Nursing Models Series). Sevenoaks: Hodder & Stoughton.

We always do it this way. *Nursing Times* 1989, **85**, (41)

22

MENSTRUATION AND ASSOCIATED PROBLEMS

The physiology of the menstrual cycle is described in Chapter 2. Menstruation is a key event in women's lives, in particular its onset, the menarche, and its cessation, the menopause (also known as the climacteric or 'change of life'). The nurse should take every opportunity to foster positive attitudes to menstruation and to dispel the old wives' tales and myths which surround it. Normal hygiene measures such as daily baths or showers are particularly important at this time and it is not normally necessary for any significant change in life-style to be made. The use of towels or tampons is usually an individual choice, and is only occasionally governed by any medical factor. Whichever method is chosen the towel or tampon should be changed every four to six hours, and women should be reminded to check for 'forgotten' tampons at the end of each period. Failure to remove the last tampon causes an offensive vaginal discharge and very occasionally is associated with toxic shock syndrome. This is an acute, severe infection which occurs suddenly and may be fatal.

The length of the menstrual cycle will vary from one woman to another, and menstruation may be expedited or delayed by stress. Variations in the length and character of the cycle also occur at the beginning of the woman's fertile years and towards the end. The duration and amount of menstrual loss also varies considerably from one individual to another. Every woman will come to recognize what is normal for her, and it is deviations from this norm which may be significant. Many women keep a record of their periods, and this is very useful when a medical history is required, in pregnancy, at the Family Planning Clinic or if the woman has a cervical smear taken.

The menstrual history is commonly summarized in medical and nursing notes as the number of days when bleeding is seen over the length of the cycle in days. For example, a woman who experiences four days' loss every 28 days would have this information recorded as 4/28.

Blood loss during menstruation may be estimated at anything from 10 to 120 ml, with an average of about 50 ml.

PREMENSTRUAL SYNDROME OR PMS

This is also known as premenstrual tension or PMT, but the condition has a variety of physical as well as psychological manifestations, so that the use of the word 'syndrome' is more appropriate.

It is a well-researched fact that in the week before the onset of the period women are more likely to be absent from work or school, make mistakes, perform badly in examinations, be involved in a road traffic accident, commit a crime or even commit suicide. The latter extremes are rare, and many women feel minimal or no disruption to their life or function, but for those who do sympathetic help is essential. The woman may feel that the female doctor or nurse is more empathetic to this problem.

Physical symptoms include breast swelling and tenderness, a 'bloated feeling' in the abdomen, skin changes such as acne, headache and tiredness.

Psychological symptoms include depression, anxiety, irritability, lack of confidence and loss of libido.

Treatment will depend on the combination of symptoms described. Pyridoxine (vitamin B6) is helpful for some women. Many women find it helpful to explain the problem to the family, enlist their help and support, use relaxation techniques and as far as possible avoid extra stress during the week before the period is expected.

AMENORRHOEA

This is described as primary or secondary.

Primary amenorrhoea

This is the failure of the menarche. If the secondary sex characteristics are also absent the girl may need detailed endocrinological investigation. The family history may reveal a familial tendency to late menarche, and the girl and her parents may be reassured and the girl reviewed at age 16–17.

If puberty appears to be progressing the girl may have an imperforate hymen, although this condition is not common. In this case she may complain of monthly abdominal pain and other period-related symptoms, but no vaginal loss. Occasionally such girls present with pain and acute urinary retention due to the blood-filled vagina swelling still further and pressing on the bladder. The term haematocolpos is used to describe the vagina filled with blood in this way. The menstrual loss may have accumulated over months, and when released will be thick and brown.

Treatment consists of incision of the hymen under general anaesthetic, releasing the vaginal contents. Antibiotics may be prescribed to prevent infection.

Secondary amenorrhoea

This is described as absence of the periods at some stage after the menarche; the commonest cause is pregnancy.

The menstrual cycle is a complicated chain of interrelated physiological events, and dysfunction of almost any of the endocrine glands may contribute to secondary amenorrhoea. Iatrogenic causes include irradiation, injected contraceptives and large doses of some drugs. It is also a symptom related to anorexia nervosa.

DYSMENORRHOEA

Dysmenorrhoea is defined as pain with menstruation. Two types, primary and secondary dysmenorrhoea, are commonly distinguished.

Primary dysmenorrhoea

Primary dysmenorrhoea is a spasmodic type of pain, occurring at the onset of the menstrual period and lasting 1–24 hours. It is most common among young girls, sometimes beginning with the menarche and fading away spontaneously around 24 years of age or following the delivery of a full-term infant. No pathology in pelvic structures is associated with this type of dysmenorrhoea. In addition to the cramps, there may be shivering, a feeling of tension, nausea, vomiting, pallor and fainting.

The aetiology remains unclear but current theory supports prostaglandins as the cause of the increased myometrial activity and subsequent pain experienced. Excessive quantities of prostaglandins are synthesised during the breakdown of the secretory endometrium.

They cause increased muscular contractions and uterine ischaemia, and are also responsible for the symptoms of nausea, vomiting and pallor by their influence on smooth muscle.

Dysmenorrhoea is also associated with ovulation, as anovulatory cycles are rarely accompanied by dysmenorrhoea. This probably explains why the first cycles are pain-free and dysmenorrhoea in some girls is synchronous with ovulation. Also, the daughters of women who have suffered dysmenorrhoea are more frequently dysmenorrhoeic. Whether this is learned or inherited is still disputed. In any case the psyche can play a role in aggravating the symptoms but is very rarely the sole explanation. A woman's personal tolerance for discomfort undoubtedly affects her response to any pain, dysmenorrhoea being no exception.

Treatment includes a kind and sympathetic approach by all members of the health team. Prostaglandin inhibitors such as acetylsalicylic acid (aspirin) and mefenamic acid (Ponstan) may be prescribed. The addition of analgesics is useful for some women and the doctor may prescribe a course of oral contraceptives. This induces anovulatory periods and may be followed by very good results. It may also be diagnostic. Should dysmenorrhoea continue, the doctor may look for other causes. In more extreme cases, surgery may be chosen. The cervix is dilated with varying success. A presacral sympathectomy or, in desperation, a hysterectomy may be done.

Nursing intervention The school and occupational health nurses commonly deal with the girl or young woman suffering from dysmenorrhoea. She may present herself in their office, or the nurse may be asked to interview the girl or woman who frequently misses school or work because of dysmenorrhoea. Frequent, severe dysmenorrhoea should always be investigated by the gynaecologist, and it is the nurse's responsibility to suggest this to the patient and assist her in obtaining this care.

In regard to general care, the patient may need instruction in the normal anatomy and physiology of menstruation. This serves to eradicate misconceptions and lessen the fear and anxiety which may be associated with her periods. She may need some instruction in menstrual hygiene so that her period does not seem distasteful and restricting. This may simply mean a switch from sanitary pads to tampons and frequent bathing. The patient may need to be encouraged to get more exercise and be sure that she is not constipated before her period.

Immediate care involves providing a sympathetic, understanding approach, a place to lie down, a blanket for warmth, application of heat to the lower abdomen and a mild analgesic. When the symptoms are relieved, the girl often continues with her work. If the patient requires medication for relief, she should be instructed to take the tablet before dysmenorrhoea becomes acute. This will prevent the symptoms and the girl or woman feels that she has some control over the events which are happening to her rather than being totally subject to them.

Secondary dysmenorrhoea

Secondary dysmenorrhoea is a constant type of pain which often starts two to three days before the period and persists well past the first day. It may continue for a day or two following the period. Pain may radiate through the abdomen into the back and down the thighs. It occurs after several years of normal painless menses and is frequently associated with pelvic pathology. The most frequent causes are tumours, inflammatory diseases, endometriosis and fixed malpositions of the uterus. It is essentially a symptom of disease.

Should the nurse be consulted by a woman describing these symptoms, the woman should be referred to a gynaecologist immediately.

MITTELSCHMERZ

This literally means 'middle pain' and is a term used to describe pain associated with ovulation and therefore occurring mid-cycle. It is usually felt only on the side of the ovary which is releasing an egg, and is fairly short-lived.

ABNORMAL UTERINE BLEEDING—DEFINITIONS

Oligomenorrhoea is unusually scanty vaginal loss at the time of normal menses. The term is also used to describe infrequent menstrual periods.

Menorrhagia is excessive bleeding at the time of normal menses.

Polymenorrhoea refers to cyclical bleeding which is normal in amount but occurs too frequently.

Epimenorrhoea is cyclic bleeding which is both excessive and too frequent.

Metrorrhagia refers to any bleeding which occurs between menstrual periods. Any bleeding *per vaginam* at any time other than normal menses is included even if it is only slight staining.

TREATMENT OF MENORRHAGIA

Until recently menorrhagia which disabled or debilitated the woman was treated by hysterectomy. The physical and psychological effects of this operation are considerable, however, and an important new treatment is currently being evaluated. Trans-cervical resection of the endometrium (TCRE) may be performed as day surgery; many cases are done under local anaesthesia. If this relatively simple procedure is used instead of hysterectomy, women with the distressing problem of menorrhagia should have a shorter wait for treatment.

DYSFUNCTIONAL UTERINE BLEEDING

True dysfunctional uterine bleeding refers to that which occurs in the presence of endocrine dysfunction rather than organic disease. It may be seen as chronic epimenorrhagia or as an episode of acute bleeding. Some episodes of haemorrhage are caused by high levels of oestrogen in the proliferative phase of the cycle. These high levels depress the hypothalamus–pituitary complex and no ovulation occurs. Because there is no ovulation, no progesterone is produced and the endometrium remains proliferative and becomes cystic. As oestrogen levels fall, usually after a six- to eight-week period of amenorrhoea, bleeding occurs. This disorder is associated with the older woman.

Other episodes of bleeding are related to fluctuating oestrogen levels produced by an imperfectly functioning hypothalamus–pituitary–ovary feedback mechanism. Follicles are stimulated to partial maturation; some oestrogen is produced but then the level falls, producing intermittent, irregular and possibly prolonged bleeding. The causes are related to immaturity or ageing of the feedback mechanism and to imbalance induced in the system by physical or psychological factors.

In most cases treatment consists of administering the combined oral contraceptives. They exert a regulating and inhibiting effect on the endometrium and feedback mechanism. Three to six cycles of hormonal therapy are usually required to reestablish the normal menstrual pattern. A dilatation and curettage may be done initially. The endometrium is scraped, a biopsy done and then hormone therapy is initiated. If required, adjunctive therapy such as iron replacement is also started. More severe cases are treated with higher and more complex doses of oestrogens and progestins, in combination or sequence. In some cases when hormone therapy does not succeed, a hysterectomy may be necessary.

POSTMENOPAUSAL BLEEDING

Any vaginal bleeding which occurs a year or more after the cessation of the periods is viewed as potentially serious. The woman is urged to seek medical advice immediately, and the condition requires full investigation.

ENDOMETRIOSIS

Endometriosis is the location of endometrial tissue outside the uterine cavity. Although the location may be varied, the most frequent locations are in or near the ovaries, the uterosacral ligaments and the uterovesical peritoneum. Extrapelvic sites may be as varied as the umbilicus, an old laparotomy scar, vulva or even lungs. The tissue responds to the hormones of the ovarian cycle and undergoes a small menstruation just like the uterine endometrium. Statistics vary, but perhaps 5% of all patients seen by the gynaecologist suffer from endometriosis.

Aetiology

Causes may be varied. Two major theories are prevalent. One concludes that small bits of endometrial tissue are forced or regurgitated back up the uterine tube and escape into the abdomen during menstruation. The other theory points out that the peritoneum and reproductive tract derive from the same early embryological tissues. Some of the tissues may be misplanted from that early time. Under sufficient stimulation, these cells respond and differentiate into a functioning endometrial tag. Rare cases seem to be caused by small pieces of endometrium being transported to other parts of the body through the lymphatics or by the blood. This seems to be true of endometrial tissue in the limbs or in lung tissue. As the ectopic endometrium menstruates, the blood collects in little cyst-like nodules which have a characteristic bluish-black look. Usually they are peasized but may be much larger. Those in the ovary and uterosacral area often attain a size of 3–6 cm. These ovarian cysts are sometimes termed 'chocolate cysts' because of the thick, chocolate-coloured material which they contain. The cysts become surrounded by fibrous tissue which makes them easy to palpate, as they feel firm and well defined. Frequently the cyst perforates and spills its sticky contents into the abdomen. The resulting irritation promotes the formation of adhesions which readily fix the ovary or the affected area to the broad ligament or other pelvic structures.

The disease is seen most frequently in the nulliparous woman, aged 30–40. It occurs more commonly in the upper economic and social groups, presumably because of less frequent and later childbearing.

Signs and symptoms

The patient may have no symptomatology, and the disease may only be discovered incidental to abdominal surgery. More commonly, the patient complains of pain. Secondary dysmenorrhoea may appear, with pain becoming severe one to two days before menstruation. The pain gradually becomes worse and may be described as 'boring'. This is due to the distension and pain of the swollen, shedding areas contained within the fibrous capsule of the cysts. The patient may also complain of backache, dyspareunia of a deep nature localized in the posterior fornix of the vagina or persistent lower abdominal pain occurring throughout the cycle. Pain may be of an acute nature, localized in the abdomen when a cyst ruptures. The gynaecologist may suspect endometriosis when a patient is infertile, since this is a common symptom of this group. Sometimes the adhesions become severe enough to cause a bowel obstruction or painful micturition.

Diagnosis is frequently confirmed on bimanual examination when firm nodular lumps are felt in the adnexa. Visualizing the typical bluish nodules may be done by culdoscopy, laparoscopy or during a laparotomy. Diagnosis is confirmed by biopsy when endometrial glands and stroma are seen microscopically.

Laparoscopy The gynaecologist may feel that direct viewing of the pelvic organs is necessary. Examination under anaesthesia involving colpotomy, culdoscopy and culdocentesis may be used but these procedures are now being replaced by laparoscopy. It provides better lighted, direct visualization of the anterior aspect of the tubes and ovaries. The procedure is done under a general anaesthetic and aseptic conditions.

To avoid damage and to obtain better visualization of the abdominal and pelvic contents, the cavity is distended by the introduction of carbon dioxide. The abdominal wall is lifted by the gas above the underlying organs. The patient is tilted head downwards to about a 45° angle, shifting the abdominal contents up and away from the site of insertion of the laparosco· and from the pelvis. Through a small incision in lower rim of the umbilicus a trocar and cannula are inserted on an angle; the trocar is then withdrawn and the endoscope inserted. It enters the peritoneal cavity approximately half-way between the umbilicus and the symphysis pubis. The contents of the abdomen and pelvis are observed and the uterus may be manipulated from below by a clamp in the cervix—this changes angles and brings the organs into better view. At the end of the procedure the endoscope is withdrawn, the gas expressed from the abdomen through the cannula and the incision closed with a clip or stitch which is removed in 24–48 hours.

There are few complications, but cardiac arrhythmias, collapse and death have been recorded. The patient may complain of some mild abdominal or shoulder pain following the procedure. This is usually abdominal gas which collects beneath the diaphragm and is not intestinal colic. The gas is absorbed gradually over a few days, but a change of position may help. Severe pain or signs of abdominal tenderness or tightness should be reported.

The patient receives pre- and postoperative care, but does not require a shave preparation. She is ambulatory on return from the recovery room and generally returns to a full diet immediately.

Treatment

This is based on the age of the patient, her desire for more children and the severity of the disease. Pregnancy relieves the symptoms and may be advised if the couple want more children. Pseudopregnancy may be achieved by the administration of progesterone for varying periods of time, or danazol 200–800 mg daily for six months.

Treatment may be surgical and is directed at preserving reproductive function. Affected areas are removed, and fixed organs released. Infertility often ceases following surgery. In severe cases a hysterectomy may be done. Depending on the extent of the cystic involvement, oophorectomy may also be performed. The symptoms usually disappear at menopause as ovarian atrophy begins and hormonal stimulation declines.

FURTHER READING

BEARD, M. (1984) *Understanding Premenstrual Tension*. London: Pan.
DALTON, K. (1971) *The Menstrual Cycle*. 2nd edn, New York: Pantheon.
GOULD, D. (1990) *Nursing Care of Women*. Prentice Hall.

23

THE MENOPAUSE

The sexual functions of the male and female continue throughout adult life. Given health and opportunity, the male's sexual and reproductive capabilities are life-long; the only major change is a slowing of sexual response and a gradual reduction in libido (sexual drive).

Women, however, present a different picture. Reproductive function, usually demonstrated by menses, continues until middle age. Then, at the average age of 50, women cease menstruating. The cessation of menstruation is perhaps the most obvious sign of menopause, or 'change of life'. Actually menopause, in onset and duration, resembles puberty, which was a gradual awakening of reproductive function over a period of six months to two years. This transitional period is known as the climacteric. The climacteric may take a few months to several years and is the result of altered ovarian function. Ovarian follicles cease to ripen. The endometrium does not respond as richly, and menstruation becomes scantier and shorter in duration. The women may have several anovulatory cycles, just as she may have had in puberty. Eventually the menses may become irregular and finally cease. Menopause is said to be complete when the woman has had no menses for one year. As the perimenopausal woman may ovulate erratically, family planning advice is important to her. She cannot assume she will not become pregnant until menopause is complete, after which the risks of pregnancy occurring are very slight.

Decreasing oestrogen levels stimulate gonadotrophic hormones (FSH, LH) which show a proportionate rise, but the ovary does not respond fully.

SYMPTOMS OF THE MENOPAUSE

Many women weather the menopause with minimal upset. However, it is a time of great change and often potential stress. It is likely to coincide with adolescent problems, children leaving home, retirement or that of her partner, elderly relatives needing care, in any combination.

'Hot flushes' This is a symptom which is often belittled, but it is very distressing and uncomfortable for many women. These episodes of flushing may last for a few seconds or up to 20 minutes. Night sweats may also occur, drenching nightclothes and disturbing sleep.

Psychological symptoms These may include depression, anxiety, forgetfulness and irritability.

Vaginal dryness and atrophy This may cause dyspareunia and loss of libido, but the use of a lubricant such as KY jelly will help. Topical application of oestrogen cream may also be prescribed. Women should be encouraged to see this problem as treatable. Nurses can do much to foster positive attitudes to sexuality in older women. Once her partner no longer has the stresses of work and the fear of unwanted pregnancy is safely past there is no reason why sex in the later years cannot be fulfilling and joyful.

Skin problems   There may be changes in skin and hair as a result of falling oestrogen levels (hence the hailing of oestrogen creams as the panacea for wrinkles).

Osteoporosis   This has been called the silent epidemic and public awareness of the problem has been very low until the late 1980s. Falling oestrogen levels lead to a steady reduction in bone structure. It is now estimated that one in four women will have suffered an osteoporotic fracture by the age of 60 years, and one in every two by the age of 70 years. One-third of female orthopaedic beds are said to be occupied by women with osteoporotic problems. Deaths resulting from osteoporosis, mainly presenting as fracture of the femoral neck in women over 70 years of age, account for more deaths per annum in the UK than those caused by carcinoma of the breast, ovary and uterus. Morbidity also includes severe pain and disability from osteoporosis of the spine. Osteoporosis is therefore emerging as a major problem of the menopause.

Cardiovascular disease   Oestrogen protects the cardiovascular system and the incidence of cardiovascular disease, cerebrovascular accidents, hypertension and raised lipid levels rises significantly in the menopause.

HORMONE REPLACEMENT THERAPY (HRT)

Perhaps because a formerly male-dominated medical profession tended to belittle the symptoms of the menopause, and to see the whole process as an integral part of women's lives which had to be endured, HRT is still regarded by some as an unnecessary extravagance.

Although it is by no means a routine treatment to be handed out to all, it has immense benefits for the woman whose symptoms are distressing. It has been shown to conserve bone structure, so delaying the onset of osteoporosis, and to reduce the risks of cardiovascular disease.

The aim of HRT is to offset the dramatic fall in oestrogen levels. Doses of oestrogen are much lower than those used in the contraceptive pill. The fear initially was of an increased risk of endometrial carcinoma, but it has now been shown that a combined regimen, with progesterone, is safe and effective.

Women must be fully informed before they start to take HRT. Unless she has had a hysterectomy the woman is at risk of endometrial carcinoma if she takes oestrogen alone. However, the effect of progesterone, which is taken for about 12 days per month in order to mimic premenopausal physiology, is to produce a withdrawal bleed. For women who are relieved not to have periods the advantages and disadvantages must be carefully balanced.

The oestrogen component of HRT may be taken orally, administered transdermally in the form of a skin patch, or as a subcutaneous implant which will be effective for several weeks. Oestrogen cream may be used topically for vaginal dryness, and oestrogen suppositories are produced, but are little used in view of the more satisfactory routes available. Progesterone is taken orally.

Many doctors now believe that all women who have had a premature menopause for any reason should have HRT, probably until the age of expected menopause, and then for about another five years. Most women who have a hysterectomy but whose ovaries are conserved will not show immediate symptoms of the menopause. However, sometimes ovarian function will fail, perhaps as a result of the blood supply being damaged during surgery.

Women with a family history of osteoporosis may be offered HRT. Bone density scans show early osteoporotic changes before symptoms arise. Ideally HRT is prescribed for these women as soon as these changes are seen. Other women at risk of developing osteoporosis are those who have Turner's syndrome, severe anorexia nervosa with amenorrhoea, thyrotoxicosis or women taking corticosteroids.

Hormone replacement therapy may be given for a few months or may be long-term. The woman is asked to visit her doctor regularly when her blood pressure will be checked; she will be offered a breast check, and a cervical smear if appropriate. Any side effects will be noted and the treatment is reviewed. HRT is not normally given to women who have had an oestrogen-dependent carcinoma in the past. Relative contraindications include endometriosis, endometrial hyperplasia, thromboembolic disease, severe varicose veins, diabetes, hypertension, fibroids and gallstones.

FURTHER READING

COOPER, W. (1976) *No Change*. London: Arrow Books.
GOULD, D. (1990) *Nursing Care of Women*. Englewood Cliffs, NJ: Prentice-Hall.
NACHTIGALL, L. & HEILMAN, J. R. (1986) *Oestrogen—the New Women's Dynamic*. London: Arlington Books.

24

CONGENITAL ABNORMALITY OF THE REPRODUCTIVE TRACT

The girl or woman who is found to have an abnormality of the reproductive tract will be shocked and will have many questions about the implications of such findings. In some cases it will be the parents of a baby girl who have to face this situation and they too will have many questions about her long-term future. They may have to make decisions about corrective surgery, and often a definite prognosis as to function and future fertility cannot be given. It is difficult for parents to accept that their child may not have full sexual and reproductive function in the future.

Questions must be answered candidly and as fully as current knowledge permits. It is wrong to give false reassurance or raise unrealistic hopes.

DEVELOPMENTAL ABNORMALITY

Although the sex of the zygote is determined genetically at fertilization obvious sex differentiation is not seen until the seventh week of intrauterine life. At this stage the genital ridge of the embryo develops into a rudimentary testis or ovary. In the female infant an elaborate bilateral duct system, the Müllerian system, develops at the same time. As the fetus grows this duct system should fuse in the midline. It is partial or complete failure of this fusion which leads to vary-

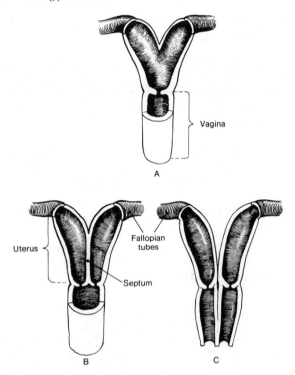

Fig. 24.1 Some abnormalities of the uterus resulting from incomplete fusion of the ducts. A, Bicornuate uterus. B, Septate uterus and a double cervix. C, Double uterus, cervix and vagina.

ing degrees of abnormality of the reproductive tract. See Fig. 24.1.

Bicornuate uterus This means 'two horns', and there is a dip in the top of the corpus or body of the uterus. This may cause habitual abortion, preterm labour or repeated breech presentation as the shape of the uterus makes cephalic presentation almost impossible. The extent of the problems caused depends on the degree of abnormality. The problem is likely to remain un-detected until pregnancy.

Septate uterus with double cervix Here the division is greater. A pregnancy may develop in either side of the uterus, but preterm labour is likely and vaginal examination during labour will show that one cervix will dilate more than the other.

Double uterus, cervix and vagina The woman with this type of abnormality is likely to present with dif-ficulties once she becomes sexually active.

Imperforate hymen This is discussed in Chapter 22 under the heading of primary amenorrhoea.

GENETIC ABNORMALITY

As fertilization occurs the zygote normally acquires either XX or XY sex chromosomes, that is female or male. Occasionally this is not the case. The result may be obvious at birth with ambiguous genitalia; alter-natively, the genitalia may appear to be male or female at birth and the child will be brought up as appropriate until puberty when a state of intersex will become apparent. In some types of intersex there is an endo-crine cause so that a girl may produce excess androgens and a boy produce too little.

It is extremely difficult for two very new parents to be told at delivery that there is uncertainty as to the sex of their child. Chromosomal studies will be carried out immediately.

Turner's syndrome In this condition there is loss of one X chromosome; the baby's sex chromosomes are shown as XO. The baby will look female at birth though there are certain physical signs which may be detected. She will fail to develop secondary sexual characteristics and will be infertile.

Klinefelter's syndrome   In this syndrome there is an extra X sex chromosome. It occurs in boys, so that the sex chromosomes are XXY. Secondary sex characteristics are incomplete and there may be breast development. These boys are also infertile.

True hermaphrodite   This is very rare and is a state of true intersex. The individual will exhibit both male and female characteristics and will be brought up as whichever sex appears dominant.

ATRESIA OF THE REPRODUCTIVE ORGANS

The vagina may have failed to develop and the uterus may also be absent. Plastic surgery is aimed at enabling the woman to be sexually active.

FURTHER READING

GOVAN, A. D. *et al.* (1985) *Gynaecology Illustrated.* 3rd edn. Edinburgh: Churchill Livingstone.
MACKAY, E. V., BEISCHER, N. A., COX, L. W., & WOOD, C. (1988) *Illustrated Textbook of Gynaecology,* W. B. Saunders.
WATSON, J. E. & ROYLE, J. R. (1987) *Watson's Medical-Surgical Nursing and Related Physiology,* 3rd edn. London: Baillière Tindall.

25

TRAUMA TO THE REPRODUCTIVE TRACT

Trauma to the reproductive tract, however caused, will be a very difficult experience for the woman or girl and she will require sensitive support. Lack of understanding and counselling at the time of injury may lead to deep-seated psychosexual problems, difficulties in relationships and much unhappiness in the future.

RAPE

The legal definitions of rape and sexual assault vary in different countries.

In the UK rape is legally defined in the 1976 Sexual Offences (Amendment) Act as 'when a man has unlawful sexual intercourse with a woman without her consent and at the time he knows that she does not consent to the intercourse or is reckless as to whether or not she consented to it.' Until 1990 in the UK there was no legal acknowledgement that rape may occur within a marriage, but this is now admissible.

Sexual intercourse in the context of rape need not involve complete penetration, but it is acknowledged as a violent and aggressive act. As such it will have a traumatic effect on the victim.

Initially the girl or woman will be in a state of shock which may present as a very calm, controlled front, but most will be very distressed. She may express disbelief, fear, anxiety, guilt, shame, helplessness or anger. These emotions may result in complaints of physical symptoms such as inability to eat or sleep, headaches, fatigue and various gynaecological symptoms. She may be fearful and anxious, particularly with regard to further attack. She may withdraw from any sexual relationship.

Society often reinforces the guilt element by suggesting that the girl's behaviour contributed to the attack. The fear of an unsympathetic hearing, and her own sense of denial may make the victim reluctant to report the offence. There is often a feeling that judges are unduly lenient with sex offenders at trial.

Following this acute phase of shock most individuals adjust and resume their normal life-style.

The majority, however, will find that the experience is revived in their memory by some life event, whether it be the anniversary of the rape, a gynaecological examination or the birth of a baby. Some women have described the similarity between a 'high-tech' birth and sexual assault and have found the experience extremely traumatic.

TREATMENT

Rape victims need sympathetic support and skilled counselling. If counselling is declined immediately after the event the woman should be assured of the availability of such help at any time in the future. The names and addresses of suitable support groups should be given to her.

Immediate physical care involves the taking of a detailed history. In the interests of justice and the protection of other women the patient should be encouraged to involve the police. (If she contacts the police before seeking medical help she will be examined by the police surgeon.) Samples are taken for forensic evidence, she is examined to determine the extent of physical injury and will be screened for pregnancy and sexually transmitted disease over the ensuing weeks. If appropriate she may be offered 'morning after' contraception.

The victim's family or friends should be included in the initial care and support given by the nurse. They should be encouraged to support the girl or woman, rather than apportioning blame or being judgemental. They should be told what support and help is available to her, and how she may react over the following weeks.

FISTULAE

Fistulae may occur between the vagina or uterus and the bladder, urethra or rectum (Fig. 25.1). They can occur as a sequel to injury during labour and delivery, surgery, and disease processes, such as carcinoma, and radiation therapy.

When urinary fistulae develop, some urine leaks into the vagina or uterus. Rectal fistulae cause the escape of flatus and faeces into the vagina. In both instances, irritation to the tissues occurs. An offensive odour develops and causes much embarrassment for the patient. Since many fistulae spontaneously heal within a matter of several weeks, treatment may be postponed. During that period nursing care is very important to the patient. Frequent perineal care is required to keep the patient clean. Cleansing and deodorizing douches may be ordered. High enemas may be given to reduce the constant flow of faeces. Care should be taken to go above the fistula with the rectal tube. If the fistula does not heal spontaneously,

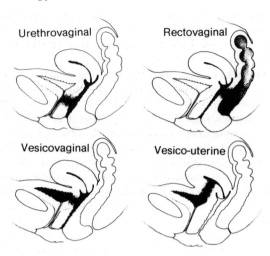

Fig. 25.1 Fistulae: urethrovaginal; rectovaginal; vesicovaginal; and vesico-uterine.

surgery may be indicated. Following surgery involving the bladder, the patient may return from the operating room with a urethral as well as a suprapubic catheter. Drainage must be maintained so that pressure on the repaired area is kept at a minimum. Repair may also include implantation of the ureters elsewhere. Rectal fistulae may be repaired and a temporary colostomy established in order to provide time to heal. Ambulation may be postponed for a few days. The woman may be discharged home on restricted activity until the doctor advises that the repair is complete.

FEMALE CIRCUMCISION

This ritual is performed on girls before puberty in certain rural parts of Africa and the Middle East. Its aim is to promote chastity before marriage and fidelity afterwards. Surprisingly it is often the women in the family who maintain and uphold this tradition, and who perform the procedure.

Excision involves cutting out the clitoris and the anterior parts of the labia; infibulation is a more extensive procedure where the operator sutures the remaining genitalia to leave a small opening for the husband to penetrate on the wedding night. The opening may be so minute that the husband has to cut it before penetration can take place. The young bride may then present in the Accident and Emergency Department mutilated and bleeding, or after a few days when infection has set in. In other cases the small child may be brought to hospital with infection following the ritual. Such children may arrive *in extremis* with septicaemia, and may die. The woman who has suffered circumcision may also be seen in the delivery room; the relatives will often resuture her genitalia when she arrives home.

The practice is deplored in the UK but is still carried out.

FURTHER READING

ASHURST, P. & HALL, Z. (1989) *Understanding Women in Distress*. London: Routledge.

IPEMA, D. K. (1979) Rape: the process of recovery. *Nursing Research*, No. 28, 272–275.

MACKAY, E. V., BEISCHER, N. A., COX, L. W., & WOOD, C. (1988) *Illustrated Textbook of Gynaecology*. W. B. Saunders.

ORR, J. (1984) Violence against women. *Nursing Times*, **80**(17), 34–36.

WATSON, J. E. & ROYLE, J. R. (1987) *Watson's Medical-Surgical Nursing and Related Physiology*, 3rd edn. London: Baillière Tindall.

26

INFLAMMATION AND INFECTIONS OF THE REPRODUCTIVE TRACT

Some genital infections are discussed in Chapter 27 since they are frequently, though not exclusively, transmitted by close sexual contact.

THE VULVA

Genital warts and herpes are discussed in Chapter 27.

Behcet's syndrome This is an ulcerative condition which may involve other systems to cause joint pains, thrombophlebitis and neurological problems.

Bartholinitis Bartholinitis is an infection of the greater vestibular gland and may or may not be gonorrhoeal in origin. The infection is an ascending one, progressing up the ducts to the gland. Symptoms are usually those of an acute infection—pain, swelling, inflammation and a purulent discharge. Cellulitis of the surrounding tissues aggravates the situation, but the infection may localize and become an abscess. This is usually excised and drained. Sometimes the infection subsides, leaving the duct scarred and occluded. This may be followed by a cyst filled with the secretions of the gland which now cannot escape. The cyst is usually a painless swelling in the lower third of the labium minus. Treatment is to excise the cyst and gland. Alternatively, a marsupialization (conversion of the duct into a pouch) of the cystic duct may be done. This leaves the functioning gland in place.

Hot baths, saline soaks and/or the use of a bidet may be ordered following surgery. The patient should be advised on frequency of bathing and how to perform adequate vulval toilet before she is discharged.

The vulva is also susceptible to any dermatological condition such as furunculosis, psoriasis, eczema or intertrigo.

Vulval pruritus is a distressing symptom and may be caused by a variety of infections or infestations, but occasionally may be a symptom of malignant or premalignant disease.

Many vulval and vaginal conditions are exacerbated by the wearing of tights or nylon underwear which make the local environment more warm and moist.

Changes occur in the vulva as women become older. The vulva generally shrinks and atrophies, and the skin becomes thin and dry.

Leukoplakia or white lesions are terms describing particular degenerative changes in the vulva where a raised area of white, thickened skin or mucosa develops. This may be a premalignant change.

THE VAGINA

Vaginal discharge is a common complaint.

Every woman will recognize her normal vaginal secretions, which will vary from one individual to another, and it is important to differentiate between this 'physiological leucorrhoea' and a pathological vaginal discharge.

Vaginal secretions have an antibacterial and lubricant function and will vary at different times in the woman's life. They increase during sexual excitement, ovulation and pregnancy, and diminish after the menopause as oestrogen levels fall.

When a woman complains of vaginal discharge it is important to ask for specific details:

Colour.
Amount—does it necessitate wearing a pad or 'pantyliner'? How often do these need to be changed?
Odour—present or not?
Soreness or itching?
Any related symptoms—these may include dyspareunia, backache, dysuria or frequency of micturition.

Trichomoniasis

This is discussed in detail in Chapter 27 since it may also affect the woman's sexual partner and both will need treating.

Candidiasis (moniliasis)

Candidiasis occurs when the vagina is invaded by the fungus *Candida albicans*. The colloquial term for this is 'thrush'. The vaginal pH is usually 5–7. Pregnant women and diabetics are predisposed because of glycosuria and the increased glycogen present in the vagina during pregnancy. Women taking the oral contraceptive pill are also more likely to develop thrush. Contamination may be from the rectum. A thick, white, curdy vaginal discharge is present which frequently causes pruritus and irritation of the vulva. The vaginal walls are reddened and covered with typical white patches. When the patches are swabbed off, bleeding may occur. Diagnosis is confirmed microscopically from a vaginal swab.

The patient is instructed in careful perineal care and hand washing to avoid reinfection and spread of the fungus to others, especially children. Nystatin or clotrimazole applied vaginally in the form of cream or pessaries achieves good results. It may be given to pregnant women.

Senile vaginitis

Because of hormonal changes following the meno-pause, the pH rises and the glycogen stores are reduced in the vagina. The vagina loses its rugae and becomes smooth and shiny. It is now more susceptible to invasion by organisms. A sticky, mucoid discharge may appear. The patient complains of a burning in the vagina, dyspareunia and pruritus of the vagina. Occasionally, the discharge is blood flecked, as areas of the vagina ulcerate and adhesions develop and tear. Severe infection is controlled by the use of systemic antibiotics or sulpha drugs. Oestrogens are administered orally or vaginally. When the vaginitis is relieved, medication is stopped, and the patient may be advised to have cleansing vinegar douches periodically.

THE CERVIX

Cervicitis

The cervix is the main barrier against ascending infections of the genital tract. As such it is exposed to many insults. The majority of these are small lacerations which occur during childbirth or injuries associated with surgery, instrumentation or venereal disease. Bacteria invade these slits in the cervix. When the cervical epithelium is damaged, the infection easily spreads to the endocervix. Congestion and oedema follow. An increase in cervical mucus results in an elevation in vaginal pH. The cells of the endocervix begin growing out around the external os. This outgrowth of cells produces a red, granular raised lesion. As the cervix is exposed to further trauma, the eroded areas become infected again and again. Chronic cervicitis results.

The symptoms vary. Usually a heavy vaginal discharge exists. The patient may notice deep dyspareunia or some bloodstained discharge following intercourse or douching.

The diagnosis depends on the characteristic appearance of the lesion. Cytological studies are usually done to distinguish cervicitis from early carcinoma. When carcinoma is ruled out, the condition is generally treated by cautery of the endocervix. After cautery the old tissue sloughs away, followed by the regeneration of the new from the outside edges of the lesion. The patient should expect a brownish discharge for one to two weeks as the old tissue sloughs away.

Often patients with cervicitis need to be taught proper perineal care. The use of strong, irritating douches should be discouraged, and perineal hygiene is stressed.

Treatment of cervical erosion

This common problem may be treated by cautery or cryosurgery; the latter is a more recently developed technique.

Following cryosurgery women are usually advised to avoid sexual intercourse for two weeks and to use sanitary towels rather than tampons for the next menstrual period. They may expect a watery or bloody vaginal discharge, often two weeks after the procedure, as the treated area sloughs.

THE BODY OF THE UTERUS

Uterine infection may occur following labour, abortion, or surgery, or it may be tuberculous. Such infection will commonly spread upwards to involve the fallopian tubes, and so is considered in more detail in the following section.

Pyometra

This means pus in the uterine cavity. The cause is usually some obstruction of the cervix such as stenosis following radiotherapy, or carcinoma.

PELVIC INFLAMMATORY DISEASE (PID)

Pelvic inflammatory disease has come to mean all ascending pelvic infections once they are beyond the cervix. Many organisms may be responsible for the symptoms. However, among the most frequent are the gonococcus and *Staphylococcus aureus*. On occasion, tuberculosis and anaerobic bacteria can be causative. Symptoms may follow labour and delivery, a criminally induced abortion, surgical procedures, contact with gonorrhoea, or cervicitis. The condition may be acute or chronic.

Signs and symptoms

The typical picture is one of a systemic infection with fever, chills, malaise, anorexia, nausea and vomiting. This is usually accompanied by lower abdominal pain which is either unilateral or bilateral. In more chronic cases, this pain is increased before and during menstruation. Pain is experienced on movement of the

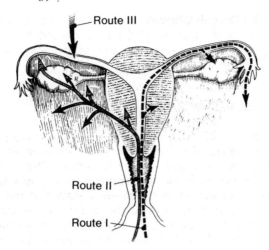

Fig. 26.1 Common routes of the spread of pelvic inflammatory disease. Route I: commonly gonococcus and staphylococcus. Route II: frequently streptococcus. Route III: tuberculosis, usually a descending infection from another source.

cervix. Leucorrhoea is present. With gonorrhoeal or staphylococcal infections the discharge is usually heavy and purulent; streptococcal infections cause a thinner, more mucoid discharge.

Spread of the infection occurs by two typical routes, which are demonstrated in Fig. 26.1. Symptoms depend on which route the infection follows. In Route I the bacteria spread along the surface of the endometrium to the tubes and into the peritoneum. The consequences of this route may be adhesions or cysts of the tube, with consequent infertility. In more advanced cases abscesses develop about the ovary or in the cul-de-sac. Infection following Route II is spread mainly through the lymphatics and produces a pelvic cellulitis in contrast to the more localized endometritis or salpingitis (infection of the uterine tube) of

Route I. Thrombophlebitis may follow this cellulitis. Advanced and virulent infections admitted by either route may become systemic and may show all the signs of septicaemia.

Treatment and nursing care

The patient with an acute episode is usually admitted to the hospital. She may or may not be isolated, depending on the cause of her infection. The patient is placed on bed-rest in semi-Fowler's position to promote drainage of pus into the vagina and the cul-de-sac. Vulval toilet should be done as needed to keep the patient clean and comfortable. Douching is usually avoided, since it may only advance the infection further. Heat to the lower back and abdomen may be soothing. Analgesics and sedation may be ordered. The patient will receive antibiotics following culture and sensitivity studies. In some cases blood cultures may be obtained. Surgical treatment is deferred, if possible, until the infection is controlled. A culdocentesis or colpotomy may be done to drain a pelvic abscess. Tubo-ovarian abscesses may require an abdominal approach. In cases of prolonged, debilitating infections which are resistant to conservative treatment, salpingectomy or hysterectomy may be done.

Chronic pelvic inflammation is a depressing condition which may inhibit the woman's life-style considerably. She may be forced to take repeated sick leave and will often feel unwell, with chronic pain. She may have to face the prospect of infertility. If this is not an apparent problem she will be advised not to have an intrauterine contraceptive device fitted.

Endometriosis is another important cause of chronic pelvic pain, but is not strictly an inflammation or infection and is discussed in more detail in Chapter 22.

FURTHER READING

BARNES, J. & CHAMBERLAIN, G. (1989) *Lecture Notes on Gynaecology*, Oxford: Blackwell Scientific Publications, 6th edn.

MACKAY, E. V., BEISCHER, N. A., COX, L. W. & WOOD, C. (1988) *Illustrated Textbook of Gynaecology*. W. B. Saunders.

WATSON, J. E. & ROYLE, J. R. (1987) *Watson's Medical-Surgical Nursing and Related Physiology*, 3rd edn. London: Baillière Tindall.

27

SEXUALLY TRANSMITTED DISEASES

The area of sexually transmitted disease is a delicate one. The person is referred to a 'special' or genito-urinary clinic where confidentiality is maintained. The patient may attend without a medical referral.

The nurse should remember that it may have been very difficult for the woman to summon the courage to attend the clinic. She may feel ashamed and guilty, apprehensive as to how she will be treated, and will wonder what the implications will be in terms of her relationships.

She will be asked detailed questions about her sexual activities over the preceding months which she may find difficult, and if she has an infection her sexual partners may have to be traced.

The most common conditions classed as sexually transmitted diseases are still gonorrhoea and syphilis. Less common ones in the UK are chancroid lympho-granuloma venereum and granuloma inguinale, which are seen more frequently in tropical countries. Other infections which are commonly spread by sexual contact include *Trichomonas*, *Candida* (Monilia), genital herpes, papilloma or wart viruses, *Chlamydia*, *Myco-plasma* and *Gardnerella vaginalis*. Infestations such as pubic lice and scabies may also be spread by sexual contact.

Most cases of sexually transmitted disease are treated on an out-patient basis, and the patient must be taught how to protect herself and others. First, the nature and transmission of the disease should be understood. No immunity develops and reinfection can occur easily. Strict personal and perineal hygiene should be observed.

These diseases may be very distressing to the patient. The patient may experience guilt feelings, and marital difficulties may arise when one partner infects the other. The disease carries a social stigma. For these reasons, confidentiality must be maintained by the nurse at all times; the issue is protected by law and the disease is reportable. Contacts must be identified and discreetly followed by the health adviser. The nurse, by explaining the nature of the disease, usually obtains the patient's cooperation in identifying contacts. In addition, the nurse should include sexually transmitted diseases in any lectures she prepares on general health education in schools so that the population may become more aware of the signs and symptoms as well as the modes of transmission of these diseases.

GONORRHOEA

The specific organism causing gonorrhoea is *Neisseria gonorrhoeae*, and it is transmitted almost exclusively by sexual intercourse. The organism dies quickly when not harboured in the human body.

Signs and symptoms   Symptoms appear two to 10 days after the initial contact.

In the adult female the vagina with its layers of squamous epithelium is resistant to the gonococcus. Therefore, the vulnerable areas are the vestibular glands, the urethra and the endocervix. The glands become red, swollen and sore. A purulent discharge may drain from the urethra and the ducts of the glands. Leucorrhoea is present in cases in which cervicitis accompanies the picture. Dysuria and frequency often occur. In about 50% of women the symptoms may be mild and vague. The infection may ascend above the cervix and may form the characteristic picture described in pelvic inflammatory disease (see Chapter 26).

Diagnosis is made on the basis of organisms seen in smears or cultures. To obtain these specimens the patient is instructed not to pass urine for approximately two hours before the cultures are taken. The vulva is not cleansed first. With the patient in a lithotomy position, smears are taken from the urethra, cervix and the ducts of the vestibular glands.

Treatment   Treatment with antibiotics, notably penicillin, is highly successful and has succeeded in reducing the incidence of complications.

In 1976 a drug-resistant strain of *Neisseria gonorrhoeae* was identified; this strain of the organism produces an enzyme (penicillinase) that inactivates penicillin. Patients infected with this resistant strain are treated with spectinomycin or a cephalosporin. Treatment is judged to be successful in cases in which repeated cultures are negative.

Hand washing following any handling of the genitalia is imperative, as the gonococcus can be readily carried to the eye, which quickly becomes infected. Blindness may ensue if treatment is not received. Women who are handling small children need to be especially careful. The vagina of a pre-pubertal girl is sensitive to the gonococcus because it lacks the protective layers of squamous epithelium. A form of vulvovaginitis may occur as a result of contamination from a family member. Sexual intercourse is to be avoided until the doctor notifies the patient she is cured. The nurse must practise all she teaches by following strict medical asepsis while caring for patients who are in the infectious stages of the disease. All equipment must be sterilized following use, and dressings or swabs are disposed of in a safe way.

NON-SPECIFIC URETHRITIS

Non-specific urethritis is an infection of the male urethra. The man complains of mild gonorrhoea-like symptoms which may become severe. It is important to rule out gonorrhoea as a cause. The onset of the symptoms is frequently related to coitus, often during menstruation when vaginal bacteria are increased, but in other cases no obvious link exists.

The infection may be due to one of several agents, but in 40% of cases is the result of a chlamydial infection. Chlamydia are a group of organisms which multiply like bacteria but do so only in the host cell, like viruses.

Cultures for *Chlamydia trachomatis* are made from swabs of the anterior urethra and from first urethral washings. Tetracycline is the treatment of choice. Those unable to take tetracycline, including pregnant women and children, are treated with erythromycin. Sexual intercourse is contraindicated during the acute stage as it prolongs the symptoms. Repeat cultures are made to confirm the effects of treatment.

In women symptoms may be few, the main one being vaginal discharge which may range from being watery to purulent. It can also contribute to non-specific cervicitis, vaginitis and pelvic inflammatory disease (PID). The newborn may acquire the infection during delivery through the vagina, sometimes causing conjunctivitis. For these reasons many doctors treat the female partners of infected men. It is hoped this will prevent later development of chlamydial related pelvic disease in these women and reduce the incidence of newborn eye and chest infections. Unlike syphilis and gonorrhoea, reporting and identification of contacts is not mandatory.

SYPHILIS

Syphilis is a more serious disease and, fortunately, is less common than gonorrhoea. The causative organism is the spirochaete *Treponema pallidum*.

Signs and symptoms Incubation varies between 10 and 90 days. In most cases the disease is spread by sexual intercourse. As with the gonococcus, the spirochaete does not survive outside the host. In the untreated condition, three stages are distinguished. The stages may overlap or be widely separated. The primary lesion is a small, painless chancre or ulcer. It is deep and has indurated edges. Usually, this chancre heals spontaneously, giving the false impression that the disease is cured. This primary lesion appears most commonly on the penis of the male. In the female, it may appear on the labia, vagina or cervix. The secondary stage is usually characterized by a rash appearing over the body. This rash may be accompanied by condylomata lata on the vulva. This is a cauliflower-like collection of flat, grey vulvar warts. As in all lesions of syphilis, these are teeming with spirochaetes and are highly infectious. The rash is usually accompanied by malaise and fever. In a short period the rash regresses and the patient enters the latent stages. Latency refers to the absence of symptoms in the infected individual. Pregnant women can still infect their fetus *in utero*, thus demonstrating the infectiousness of the blood. However, progress of the disease in the individual seems arrested and only rarely can others be infected in this stage. Three outcomes are now possible: (1) the patient proceeds immediately or after a delay of 10–30 years to the third stage; (2) the disease remains latent for the rest of the person's life; or (3) a spontaneous cure occurs. In the tertiary stage the bones, heart, and central nervous system, including the brain, can be affected. Personality disorders arise and the typical ataxic gait of the tertiary syphilitic appears. A large, ulcerating necrotic lesion known as a gumma now occurs. Rarely is it seen in the genital tract, but it may occur on the vulva or in the testes. At this stage the disease may be arrested but not reversed.

Diagnosis is made by a careful history, clinical findings, and cultures or biopsies from the lesions. Blood serology is also assessed. Since blood serology is not positive for about four weeks after the onset of the disease, the early diagnosis is made from scrapings of the lesions. They can be seen on dark-field examination. These scrapings are made before antibiotic therapy is initiated so that the diagnosis can be confirmed.

Treatment Treatment is by antibiotic, and penicillin is the drug of choice. A series of injections is necessary; oral medication is not effective. The Jarisch–Herxheimer reaction is a local and systemic reaction which may occur after beginning antisyphilitic therapy. Fever, sweating and headache appear two to 12 hours after treatment. The reaction should be differentiated from a penicillin reaction.

In syphilis, the disease may be transmitted by direct contamination with living spirochaetes of a laceration. For this reason, the nurse who has a break in her skin must be very careful when dealing with the lesions of syphilis. Gloves should be worn. Once therapy has been initiated, the patient is usually non-infectious within 48 hours.

CHANCROID

Chancroid is caused by a gram negative organism. It produces a painful, soft chancre or ulcer. The inguinal lymph glands are swollen and painful.

Treatment consists of a course of sulphafurazole or a broad-spectrum antibiotic.

LYMPHOGRANULOMA VENEREUM

This disease is caused by one of the *Chlamydia* group of organisms. Its first manifestation is a small papule or vesicle which appears one to two weeks after infection; one to two weeks later this develops into an ulcer which may cause some pain. After a further two to three weeks there is inguinal adenitis. These nodes may be multiple and adherent; the mass may break down into multiple sinuses.

The condition is treated with a course of tetracycline, erythromycin or sulphafurazole.

GRANULOMA INGUINALE

This condition is caused by one of the *Klebsiella* group of organisms. The first symptom is a painless nodule which progresses to form an ulcer. This may become extensive, involving the vulva and perianal area. It causes vaginal discharge, dyspareunia and local swelling.

Treatment consists of a two to three week course of tetracycline or erythromycin.

TRICHOMONIASIS

This condition is caused by a protozoon, *Trichomonas vaginalis*, which causes a typical grey, yellow or greenish frothy vaginal discharge. The woman will complain of soreness and dyspareunia.

Metronidazole is given to treat both partners.

CANDIDIASIS (MONILIASIS)

This is discussed in more detail in Chapter 26 as it is a common problem for women generally. However, it often infects the woman's sexual partner, in which case both will need treatment.

GENITAL HERPES

Genital herpes is commonly caused by herpes simplex virus II (HSV II) and oral herpes by HSV I. However, oral sex may complicate this picture and the viruses interchange. The incubation period may be days or weeks; initial symptoms include burning, itching and hyperaesthesia of the vulva. Tender papules and vesicles then develop and the patient may complain of malaise, headache, neuralgia and acute dyspareunia.

This is a distressing complaint which tends to recur. Like oral herpes it is often exacerbated by stress and sunlight.

HSV may be fatal for the neonate, and a woman with active herpes at term may need to be delivered by caesarean section.

Women who have suffered from genital herpes are advised to have annual cervical smears as HSV is thought to predispose to carcinoma of the cervix.

Topical and systemic antiviral agents may be of some use.

GENITAL WARTS

The genital wart virus is one of the human papilloma virus (HPV) group. The other name for the condition is condylomata acuminata. The incubation period is weeks or months. The initial wart 'seeds' locally, flourishing in the warm moist conditions, and infection or ulceration may occur. The warts may spread to the vagina and cervix.

The woman who has suffered from HPV infection is advised to have annual cervical smears as there appears to be a correlation between wart virus and carcinoma of the cervix. Indeed a previous infection may be suspected from the cervical smear, as it produces typical cell changes.

Treatment may be local application of podophyllin (not in pregnancy), cautery, cryosurgery or laser therapy.

MYCOPLASMA

Mycoplasma infects the vagina and cervix and may cause infertility.

Treatment is with tetracycline.

GARDNERELLA

Gardnerella causes a greyish-white vaginal discharge which may be frothy and slightly offensive. The woman may also complain of frequency of micturition, dysuria and pruritus.

Both partners are treated with metronidazole.

PUBIC LICE

The pubic louse, *Pediculus pubis* or crab louse, is easily conveyed to a new host by sexual contact or by sleeping in infected bedding.

Like the head louse the pubic louse bites the host to suck blood and lays eggs—nits—which adhere to the pubic hair. The bites cause intense irritation.

The specific treatment is malathion or benzyl benzoate in lotion or shampoo form. Bedding should be washed in the hot cycle of the washing machine.

SCABIES

The scabies mite, *Sarcoptes scabiei*, burrows under the skin to lay its eggs. This causes intense irritation and a fine line may be seen on the skin surface, delineating the route of the burrow. Infection secondary to scratching is common. Infestation is not confined to the genital area.

It is treated with two applications of benzyl benzoate 24 hours apart, preferably after a hot bath. Clean clothes should then be put on and all clothing and bedding washed in the hot cycle of the washing machine.

FURTHER READING

BARLOW, D. (1979) *Sexually Transmitted Diseases—the Facts*. Oxford University Press.

KING, A., NICOL, C. & RODIN, P. (1980) *Venereal Diseases*, 4th edn. London: Baillière Tindall.

OATES, J. K. (1983) *Herpes—the Facts*. Harmondsworth: Penguin Books.

THIN, R. N. (1982) *Lecture Notes on Sexually Transmitted Diseases*. Oxford: Blackwell Scientific Publications.

28

WOMEN AND AIDS

SOME DEFINITIONS

The acronym AIDS stands for acquired immune deficiency syndrome.

HIV stands for human immunodeficiency virus.

ARC stands for AIDS related complex, but this term is now less widely used.

It is important to consider the impact of AIDS on women since it is no longer a distant phenomenon affecting other people. AIDS is still popularly viewed as a 'gay' disease, but the epidemic among gay men was in fact only the first wave of the disease. The second wave arose among the drug-abusing population where needles were shared. It is now a disease affecting heterosexual individuals with almost anyone being at risk unless they can be confident that they have enjoyed a monogamous relationship with a monogamous individual neither of whom have been exposed to any risk factors. Thus more women are being infected in the UK in the early 1990s. Many of these women are infected as a result of sharing needles when abusing drugs.

An infected woman may also have to face the possibility of transmitting AIDS to her unborn child or to make the difficult decision whether or not to have a baby, and of course many women are the carers who have to face the loss of a child or sexual partner. Some of these dependants will be haemophiliacs or recipients of other infected blood products which were used before present-day screening, and they and their carers still have to face the stigma, mistrust and misinformation which remain prevalent. Similarly, some infected individuals will have contracted the disease from a single incident or may have had a brief excursion into drug misuse many years previously.

The human immunodeficiency virus causes its devastation by progressively undermining the immune system. It causes a range of infections of which AIDS is the most serious manifestation. It is important to understand that an individual may have HIV antibodies on serological testing, that is be HIV positive, but not have AIDS. Such an individual may never develop AIDS, the syndrome may develop after as long as 10 years, or the disease may progress very rapidly.

Because the serological test is for antibodies, and these are not manufactured immediately the virus enters the system it is also possible for an individual to receive a negative result to the test but already be infected. The process of producing antibodies is known as seroconversion and this may not occur until three months after infection.

COUNSELLING

It is important that women receive skilled and informed counselling before they or their family members or partners are tested for HIV.

At the time of writing individuals may be stigmatized by being tested; they may be unable to obtain a mortgage or life insurance whatever the test result since they are deemed to be at risk because they requested a test.

All individuals should be advised to practise 'safe sex' whether or not they may be infected, so that knowing a test result should not affect an individual's behaviour in this respect. Knowing one is HIV positive gives no assurance as to outcome and may cause more anxiety than it allays. However, for some the uncertainty will cause the greater degree of anxiety and this must be explored in pre-test counselling.

For both women and men it may be important because of decisions about childbearing although it is much more likely that the woman, rather than the man, will infect the child. Most people will want to consider the possibility of early death before starting a family.

MEANS OF TRANSMISSION

Infection with HIV occurs as a result of exchange of certain body fluids of which the most important is blood.

Male to female transmission is the more common form of heterosexual spread, with HIV present in the semen, but the woman is only likely to acquire the infection if she has some kind of lesion such as genital sores or a cervical erosion. If the woman passes on the infection she is probably more likely to do so if intercourse takes place during menstruation. Although vaginal intercourse is only likely to be a problem if blood is passed from the infected partner or if infected body fluids pass into the other partner's blood stream, safe sexual practices should always be followed. Nurses should be aware of these and be ready to advise.

Any form of anal intercourse, where tissue damage is likely, is classed as 'high risk'; hence the rapid spread in earlier years in the male homosexual population. It is now recognized that there is a similar risk among lesbians if one partner has had intercourse with an infected male.

Another cause of spread of the disease has in the past been from donor semen for artificial insemination by donor. Official sperm banks should now screen their clientele by careful history taking and by testing donors for HIV. Semen is then frozen for three months and another serological test is performed. Women who acquire semen from friends for self-insemination, particularly among the gay population, should be aware that this is a potentially unsafe practice.

Blood is the most infective of the body fluids; semen, vaginal secretions, urine and faeces present a moderate degree of risk; saliva and breast milk probably represent minimal or no risk.

'SAFE SEX'

Low risk sexual behaviour This includes any non-penetrative activities such as kissing, cuddling, mutual masturbation, massage. These become less safe if either partner has cuts or sores on the fingers or lips, and body fluids are exchanged.

Medium risk sexual behaviour This includes any form of vaginal, oral or anal sex using a condom, barrier or glove as necessary to prevent exchange of body fluids.

High risk sexual behaviour This is penetrative sex with no condom or barrier especially where blood is exchanged.

Condoms used should be impregnated with the spermicide nonoxynol-9 which is thought to have some effect against the virus. A water-based lubricant such as KY jelly should also be used, since others such as Vaseline may damage the rubber.

SYMPTOMS OF AIDS

When the individual who is HIV positive develops AIDS he or she is prone to opportunistic infections from organisms which are not normally pathogenic, or only mildly so. Two classic examples of this are *Pneumocystis carinii* pneumonia (PCP) and Kaposi's sarcoma (KS). Both are rare conditions outside the AIDS scenario and indeed *Pneumocystis carinii* is not regarded as a pathogenic organism.

The generalized symptoms of AIDS include the following:

Persistent generalized lymphadenopathy (PGL).
Profound fatigue lasting weeks.
Unexplained fever associated with chills and night sweats.
Unexplained weight loss of more than 10 lb in ap-proximately two months.
Thrush—oral or genital—and usually very severe and distressing.
Persistent diarrhoea.
Shortness of breath with a dry cough.
Pink or purple blotches on the skin.

AIDS AND PREGNANCY

While sexual partners and close contacts can be pro-tected from HIV infection to some extent, the unborn baby is vulnerable to transplacental infection. It is thought that some babies are not infected until de-livery. Still others are born unaffected.

It is possible that the woman who is HIV positive who becomes pregnant is at greater risk of developing AIDS. She then has to face the fact that she may not live to see her child grow up and may spend much of her life unwell. She may decide to take this risk in the hope of a cure being discovered.

No firm evidence exists as yet as to whether or not breast milk is a source of infection. There have been no proven cases of infection by this route but some authorities advise against breast-feeding.

ADVICE TO SUFFERERS

Adopt a life-style which includes a healthy diet, reduced stress and plenty of rest.

Avoid unnecessary infection and unhygienic conditions.

Cover cuts with waterproof plaster.

Avoid sharing toothbrushes and razors.

Adopt safe sexual practices in order to avoid other sexually transmitted diseases as well as to prevent the spread of the virus.

Avoid drugs which further depress the immune system.

Avoid vaccinations unless the doctor is aware of the infection.

Wash the hands after handling pets, particularly after cleaning out cages or emptying litter trays.

Blood and organ donation is not possible.

Beware of charlatans offering false advice and hope.

ADVICE TO CARERS

Wear gloves when handling body fluids.

Mop up spills of blood, urine or faeces with a solution of one part of household bleach to 10 parts of water.

Wash clothes stained with body fluids in the washing machine using the hottest wash cycle.

Burn sanitary towels, tampons or dressings or dispose of them in sealed plastic bags. There may be local problems with disposal of clinical waste and local authority personnel may need advice. Infection control staff at the local hospital will help here.

The person suffering from AIDS will experience a variety of emotions which may include depression, anger, guilt, and confusion over sexuality. He or she may feel isolated and very alone. The nurse should do as much as possible to engender positive attitudes and to educate whenever the opportunity arises. There are many popular myths, often fed by the media, which need to be exploded.

The individual suffering from AIDS is entitled to high quality nursing care without prejudice, and should be treated with respect. Nurses and doctors should take all the prescribed precautions when dealing with the body fluids of any patient. This is a safeguard for themselves, but will also help the patient with AIDS to feel less stigmatized, isolated or 'unclean'. The patient is only nursed in a single room if this is what she prefers or if there is a true risk of infection to herself or others.

FURTHER READING

DANIELS, V. G. (1985) *AIDS the Acquired Immunodeficiency Syndrome.* MTP Press.

KIRKPATRICK, B. (1988) *AIDS—Sharing the Pain.* London: Darton, Longman & Todd.

KUBLER-ROSS, E. (1969) *On Death and Dying.* New York: Macmillan.

PRATT, R. (1986) *AIDS—A Strategy for Nursing Care.* London: Edward Arnold.

TERRENCE HIGGINS TRUST (1987) *Women and AIDS.* 3rd edn.

29

TUMOURS OF THE REPRODUCTIVE TRACT

It is important to remember that many tumours, or new growths, in the female genital tract are benign. The woman who discovers that she has such a tumour may find it hard to believe, and may need much reassurance.

POLYPS

Polyps are common benign growths occurring mainly in the endometrium and cervix. The polyp has a characteristic smooth, shiny surface and is pink to deep red in colour. They are small in size, seldom exceeding more than 3 cm in length. The cause is unknown. No symptoms are usually present, but occasionally post-coital bleeding occurs. Treatment is by surgical excision of cervical polyps and may be followed by dilatation and curettage to remove endometrial polyps.

MYOMAS OF THE UTERUS

A myoma (fibromyoma, leiomyoma) is a benign tumour of the uterus composed of myometrium and fibrous tissue. Colloquially, myomas are known as 'fibroids'. At least 25% of women over 35 years of age show some evidence of myomas. The cause is unknown, but oestrogen stimulation is thought to play a part.

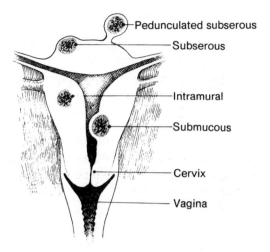

Fig. 29.1 Uterine myomas.

Myomas occur mainly in the uterine body. According to their position they are classified as subserous, submucous and intramural (Fig. 29.1), and may become pedunculated. A pedunculated fibroid in the uterine cavity may be referred to as a fibroid polyp. This may be extruded through the cervix and may come to lie in the vagina. Myomas in the broad ligament or cervix are recorded, but these locations are rare. Several fibroids of varying sizes may be present in any one uterus. As the fibroids become larger, their blood supply may be reduced, causing some degeneration. The most common is a hyaline degeneration in the middle of the myoma. This causes a loss of cellular structure and, in extreme cases, a collection of gelatinous fluid lies at the centre. Sometimes the tumour shows signs of fatty changes and may even become calcified (womb-stone). A so-called red degeneration may occur, usually in association with pregnancy. The tumour looks like raw beef on the inside. The patient shows signs of malaise with fever, rapid pulse and pain over the fibroid. Following menopause all myomas atrophy and show slight shrinkage.

Signs and symptoms

Symptoms vary with the size and location of the tumour. Frequently, with small tumours, there are no symptoms. Occasionally menorrhagia occurs. Pain is rarely a symptom but most frequently is associated with torsion of a pedunculated myoma. Sometimes the myoma passing through the cervix causes cramps. Dysmenorrhoea may occur as a result of mechanical interference. Large myomas can cause frequency or retention of urine. Pressure on veins, lymphatics, and nerves of the pelvis may cause varicosities, unilateral or bilateral oedema of the lower extremities, or a radiating pain through the thighs. Occasionally, these tumours may be the cause of abortions or infertility. Some tumours become infected.

Treatment

Treatment depends on the age of the woman, her desire for more children and the size of the myoma. In the young woman who wishes children, a myomectomy is usually done. This is the enucleation of the myoma, but the uterus is preserved. Blood loss during the operation may be extensive as the surgeon excises multiple myomas from a large uterus which may not contract efficiently. Persistent oozing of blood may occur postoperatively for the same reasons. The nurse should be alert to this possibility. In cases of very large myomas the treatment is hysterectomy.

In the young woman, myomas are not a contraindication to pregnancy and usually cause no difficulty.

Rarely, they may obstruct labour or cause a postpartum haemorrhage.

TUMOURS OF THE OVARY

Tumours of the ovary are many and varied. The aetiology of most is unknown. For purposes of clarity they are roughly divided into non-neoplasms and neoplasms. Only a few are described in each group.

Non-neoplasms

Non-neoplasms are usually simple cysts or collections of fluid surrounded by a thin capsule. They do not grow but expand only as more fluid accumulates. These physiological cysts are seen mainly during the reproductive years. The follicular cyst is the most common of this group. Corpus luteum cysts may occur as well. Theca lutein cysts develop under the stimulation of high levels of chorionic gonadotrophins.

Occasionally, the Stein–Leventhal syndrome or polycystic disease of the ovary occurs. The syndrome appears in the late teens and early twenties with variable symptoms. These may include a history of sterility, secondary amenorrhoea, hirsutism and cysts bilaterally in the ovary. The ovary shows some enlargement and presents a glistening white appearance. Microscopically, many atretic follicular cysts are present. The syndrome is thought to follow an endocrine imbalance, probably arising in the ovary but affecting the hypothalamus. The ovaries produce an excessive amount of androgens which inhibit maturation of a follicle with subsequent disturbance of the ovarian–hypothalamic relationships. What triggers the imbalance is unknown. Medical treatment consists of a course of the drug clomiphene, with or without gonadotrophins, to produce a luteinizing hormone (LH) surge and ovulation. Surgical treatment is known as a wedge resection of the ovary. About half the ovarian tissue is removed in a wedge shape. This reduces the amount of tissue producing high androgen levels, which subsequently fall and ovulation takes place. Medical treatment appears to be replacing surgical treatment.

Neoplasms

Pseudomucinous cystadenomas are the single most common neoplasms, occurring in about 40% of patients with a neoplastic ovarian growth. They may attain the largest size of any ovarian tumour. The tumour is characterized by multiple pockets filled with a thick fluid called pseudomucin. They may be bilateral and may become malignant.

Serous cystadenoma is the second most common of this group and appears to arise from germinal epithelium. The cyst contains a serous fluid. These cysts are frequently bilateral and often become malignant.

The dermoid cyst or teratoma may be cystic or solid. When it is soft, the cyst is filled with sebaceous material, hair and ordinary skin. The solid cyst frequently contains cartilage, bone, teeth, thyroid, and similar material. Rarely is the cyst malignant. It occurs most frequently in young women and may be bilateral.

Neoplasms of the ovary may also be divided into those which have some hormonal effect and those which do not. One tumour with no hormonal effect is a *dysgerminoma*. It arises from the primitive germ cells and is usually malignant. A *fibroma* is a benign solid neoplasm occurring most frequently in the post-menopausal patient. The fibroma arises from connective tissue in the ovary and may be associated with Meigs' syndrome, which is characterized by ascites and pleural effusion.

Those tumours which have hormonal effects may be further subdivided into feminizing and virilizing lesions. The most common of the rare feminizing tumours is the *granulosa cell tumour*. The tumour produces oestrogen and may induce precocious puberty or cause hypermenorrhoea or postmenopausal bleeding. It may be malignant or may be associated with carcinoma of the endometrium. The most common of the even rarer masculinizing tumours is *arrhenoblastoma*. By the production of androgens, presumably from the primitive male cell elements in the ovary, the woman is masculinized. In about 15–25% of cases it proves to be malignant.

CARCINOMA OF THE OVARY

Primary carcinoma of the ovary is usually the common adenocarcinoma. However, a review of ovarian growths is indicated, as almost any one of them has the potential to become malignant. The most common malignancy arises from the serous cystadenoma. Only one ovary may be affected but the other quickly follows, apparently because of the close lymphatic connections. About 5% of all cancers in the female arise in the ovary.

Secondary tumours represent metastases from almost any other cancer. The Krukenberg tumour deserves mention. In this case bilateral, equal involvement is usually secondary to tumours in the stomach. Back-up of the lymphatic drainage appears responsible for this particular tumour, especially since other metastases usually occur later.

Signs and symptoms

The ovarian tumour in its early stages is often symptomless. At regular yearly check-ups, palpation of the adnexa will reveal a mass. Often this may be the first discovery of the tumour. The symptoms result from the size of the tumour or its position. An increase in girth may be noticed but ignored. Pressure on the bladder causes frequency or a feeling of fullness. Constipation, oedema of the legs, anorexia and a full feeling in the abdomen may be present. Pain may be associated with stretching of the tissues as the tumour enlarges. Ascites may be present, accompanied by difficulty in breathing.

Treatment

Because of the danger of malignant growth, any ovarian mass is observed suspiciously. A rule of thumb says that any soft mass below 5 cm may be watched closely for two to three months. If no further growth occurs, then conservative treatment may be considered. Other tumours demand biopsy, and a laparotomy is indicated. Following diagnosis, the surgeon strives to preserve as much ovarian function as is possible. In premenopausal women benign growths, if size permits, will be enucleated and ovarian function preserved. Malignant growths are treated with total hysterectomy and bilateral salpingo-oophorectomy (removal of the tubes and ovaries). Surgery is followed by chemotherapy. Unfortunately, many malignancies have metastasized before discovery of the tumour. Prognosis is poor and surgery may be only palliative. Further treatment is directed toward relieving the symptoms of the terminally ill patient. Recurrent ascites may be a problem, and frequent paracentesis may be indicated.

Complications of ovarian tumours

Torsion or twisting of the growth on its stalk frequently occurs. Circulation is impeded, and necrosis may

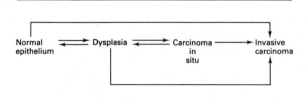

Fig. 29.2   Patterns of development of cancer of the cervix.

follow. The patient usually feels a sudden severe pain in the lower abdomen. Treatment is by excision of the tumour at an immediate laparotomy.

The cyst may rupture. Often the 'chocolate cyst' of endometriosis ruptures and drains fluid into the abdomen. Again the patient may present with an 'acute abdomen'.

Haemorrhage and infection occur in tumours as well. They are more common in the malignant tumour.

Postsurgical menopause is the result of a bilateral oophorectomy. The symptoms are similar to those of the regular menopause, but may be more severe because of the sudden withdrawal of hormones. Replacement therapy with oestrogens may begin before the patient leaves the hospital if it is not contraindicated by malignancies which are aggravated by oestrogens.

CARCINOMA OF THE CERVIX

Carcinoma of the cervix is a common malignancy in women. The woman who has borne children or had an early sex life with several partners is more apt to develop the disease.

Cancer of the cervix is a complex disease which is preceded by several earlier cervical changes (Fig. 29.2).

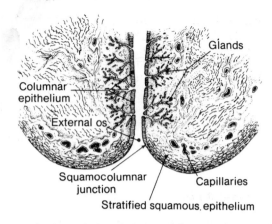

Columnar epithelium
External os
Glands
Squamocolumnar junction
Capillaries
Stratified squamous epithelium

Fig. 29.3   Squamocolumnar junction of the cervix.

These changes usually occur at the squamocolumnar junction of the cervix (Fig. 29.3), and initially are evident only on histological examination. They reflect a varied pattern of development. Some cases arise with no known precursor stage, while others appear to have gone through all the changes or any combination of them. The earlier changes may be reversible, and so do not always herald cancer. How many of these will reverse is unknown, but about 50% of women with carcinoma in situ are thought to develop invasive cancer; this development may take an average of 10 years. The cervical smear is the best method of early detection of these changes. Combined with treatment of these changes it is largely responsible for the declining mortality rates associated with cervical cancer.

Because five-year survival rates are excellent in those cases which are discovered early, the Royal College of Nursing and the Royal College of Obstetricians and Gynaecologists both recommend that all women who are sexually active or over 25 should have cervical smear tests at least every three years. The nurse has a responsibility to disseminate this knowledge. The nurse emphasizes the hopeful aspects of cure following cases of early recognition. This may encourage more women to seek medical attention by reducing their anxiety. Fear of what she may discover often seems to prevent the patient from consulting her doctor. The nurse should do her utmost to persuade the woman complaining of irregular bleeding to seek medical attention immediately.

Signs and symptoms

A small lesion develops which, in the early stages, can be confused with other cervical conditions. The early stages may be asymptomatic, but eventually some bleeding from the vagina occurs. An unusual vaginal discharge may be present which may have an offensive odour. Pain is a late symptom and is followed by weight loss, anorexia and cachexia.

Carcinoma of the cervix is divided into stages. Stage 0 is carcinoma in situ, or focal carcinoma. There is an intact basement membrane containing the malignant cells. Stage I is invasive cancer, which means that the basement membrane has been breached and the cells are invading the surrounding tissue. Stages IA and IB refer to degrees of this invasion which is still within the confines of the cervix. Unfortunately, about 20% of Stage I will already have spread to the lymphatics. A small lesion similar to an erosion may be present on the cervix. In Stage II the carcinoma has spread to close adjacent structures, and the upper third of the vagina may be involved. By Stage III invasion has reached the pelvic walls and lower vagina. Stage IV is marked by extensive pelvic involvement, including the bladder or bowel, and distant metastases may be present.

Treatment

Treatment is usually guided by the stage assigned to the situation by the gynaecologist. Since the main method of diagnosing Stage 0 carcinoma is the cervical smear test, the results of this test help to guide treatment. The smear results are organized into five classes. In Classes I and II the cells are non-malignant, and no treatment is necessary. Class III is suspicious and arouses concern. The patient is asked to have repeat smears done in three months or a biopsy is performed. Classes IV and V are positive, indicating that definite changes are present which require biopsy.

Biopsy A *punch biopsy* may be done with special punch biopsy forceps. Because of the paucity of nerve endings in the cervix, the biopsy may be done with relative comfort for the patient. She may feel something like a pinch when the biopsy is taken. A Schiller test can be done. Normally the cervix contains glycogen. This is depleted in areas of abnormal cell change. When Lugol's solution (iodine in potassium iodide) is swabbed on the cervix, the normal epithelium stains a dark brown. Glycogen-deficient areas are a pale colour by contrast, and these are the areas requiring biopsy.

Further treatment may be a *cone biopsy*. It is an operative procedure in which a cone-shaped segment of the central cervix is removed. The internal os remains intact (Fig. 29.4). On examination the section may contain all of the malignant area. In these cases the biopsy may be considered sufficient treatment. Pre- and postoperative care for the patient is similar to other vaginal surgery such as a D & C. The major difference is that these patients face the threat of a malignant disease and may be extremely anxious. Considerable skill in providing supportive nursing will be demanded of the nurse. Haemorrhage is a threat, and the patient should be warned of this. Bleeding from the biopsy site may

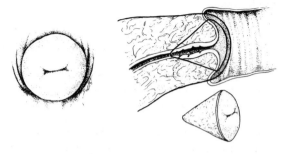

Fig. 29.4 Cone biopsy of the cervix.

occur up to a week after the biopsy when the patient is at home. The nurse should inform the patient of this possibility before discharge so that she will notify her doctor and not be unduly alarmed. Sometimes the haemorrhage is severe enough to necessitate re-admission to hospital and a blood transfusion.

The biopsy results may indicate normal cells, dysplasia, carcinoma in situ or invasive carcinoma. Many situations contribute to dysplasia, and the patient is usually treated for these and followed closely with repeat cervical smears. Some of these will revert back to normal epithelium. If they do not, a cone biopsy may be performed or, in the older woman, a hysterectomy. Carcinoma in situ may be treated with a cone biopsy if the woman wishes more children or by total hysterectomy. All carcinoma in situ must be treated to ensure prevention of invasive carcinoma. Invasive carcinoma of the cervix will be treated according to the stage in which it is classified.

Laser therapy An important advance in the treatment of Stages I–III is laser therapy. The acronym LASER stands for Light Amplification by the Stimulated Emission of Radiation. The laser beam may be directed very accurately at the precancerous lesion. The cells in the path of the beam are heated rapidly, the water within them vaporizes, and the cell bursts.

This procedure is performed under local anaesthesia in many cases, and appears to be safe and effective.

Surgery and radiation therapy   Stages IA and IB and some early Stage II's are treated by radical surgery (modified Wertheim's hysterectomy), which attempts to eliminate the cancer, and radiation therapy. There is much debate over the optimum approach. Some prefer radiation alone; others prefer surgery with or without radiation. In major medical centres, with highly qualified surgeons and sophisticated radiation equipment and radiologists, higher cure rates have been recorded with a combination of surgery and radiation. In smaller centres lacking highly experienced surgeons some quote higher cure rates for radiation alone. Most seem to agree that Stages III and IV are best treated by radiation and some palliative surgery. In cases where the surgeon feels that the tumour is surgically excisable a pelvic exenteration is done. Surgery is used in cases of a radioresistant tumour.

The patient who is having a total hysterectomy (Fig. 29.5) for carcinoma in situ will have the uterus, cervix and upper third of the vagina removed. The ovaries are usually conserved in the premenopausal woman but may be removed in the older woman. The patient is prepared as for abdominal surgery. A perineal shave preparation may be ordered as well, and the mons pubis, vulva, perineal body, and the upper third of the thighs are shaved. Postoperatively, any vaginal discharge must be observed. Some staining may occur from the vaginal cuff. A Foley catheter may be inserted and may remain in place for one or two days postoperatively. The nurse is alert to possible signs of hormonal imbalance following removal of the ovaries as well as signs of a urinary tract infection and thromboemboli.

In a Wertheim's hysterectomy, the uterus, ovaries,

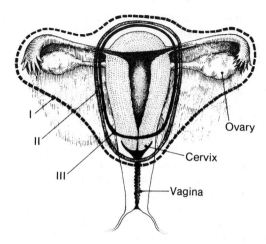

Fig. 29.5 Types of hysterectomy. I, Total hysterectomy with bilateral salpingo-oophorectomy. II, Total hysterectomy. III, Subtotal hysterectomy.

broad ligaments, surrounding tissue, upper half of the vagina and pelvic lymph nodes are removed. Sometimes the ovaries will be retained, especially in a younger woman. In a more extensive Wertheim's operation, the pelvic fascia and further lymph tissue will be removed. Preoperatively the patient has a cystoscopy examination and her ureters are catheterized. This allows them to be easily identified during the extensive pelvic dissection. The patient's vagina and cervix are painted with an iodine solution to identify any glycogen-deficient areas which would indicate further vaginal resection.

Nursing care

When the patient returns to the ward she will require general postoperative care. Two Redivac drains may have been inserted, one in each lower quadrant, and attached to a drainage system. These are removed when there is no drainage. Drainage is usually more extensive if no radiation has been given before surgery, and less if radiation has been given. Occasionally two rubber drains, one on either side, may be draining into the vagina. They are shortened about the third postoperative day and removed about the fifth day if drainage has ceased. If oozing of blood was a problem during surgery, the pelvis may have been packed with a gauze pack, the tail of which is brought out through the vaginal cuff into the vagina. This is usually shortened after 48 hours and removed in 72 hours. The ureters and bladder have been handled during surgery and may be atonic. Care must be taken to see that the catheter is draining properly and that bladder distension does not occur. The catheter should drain clear urine. Observations are made for signs of thromboemboli postoperatively; the femoral areas as well as the calves are examined. Early ambulation is encouraged, but does not merely mean sitting in a chair by the bedside for extended periods of time. Better venous return is achieved by having a patient lie in bed with her legs elevated to about 15° than by sitting for long periods of time in a chair at the bedside. Ambulation refers to movement—getting up to sit in a chair for 10–15 minutes, back to bed with feet slightly elevated, getting up to walk to the bathroom, getting up to eat lunch and back to bed to rest. Leg exercises, coughing and deep breathing are important in promoting good circulation.

Fistula formation is a hazard and the risk is greater if radiation therapy has been given prior to surgery. Because these fistulae are a result of poor blood supply and the sloughing of tissue they are a later development, usually appearing in the second postoperative week. The most common are vesicovaginal and ureterovaginal. Thus, any unusual drainage of urine must be noted. In addition, any unexplained fever or lower quadrant or flank pain should alert the nurse. The fistula is usually not repaired immediately, but postponed until a more favourable time.

A pelvic exenteration includes all of the Wertheim's hysterectomy plus a total vaginectomy and removal of portions of the bladder or bowel, depending upon the spread of the disease. The patient may return postoperatively with an ileostomy, a colostomy or an ileal conduit. In these operations preoperative bowel preparation is performed. Postoperatively, drains may be left in areas of node dissection to prevent the pooling of blood and serum which may easily lead to infection. The drains may be draining freely or may be attached to suction. Usually they are shortened daily and removed by the fifth postoperative day.

The postoperative adjustment to life may be difficult. Preoperative discussions with the doctor and nurse should help to prepare the patient. In pelvic exenteration sexual function of the vagina is lost; in a Wertheim's operation it may have to be modified. Menopause may occur as oestrogen therapy is frequently contraindicated. The care of the colostomy or ileostomy must be learned and accepted. The patient will require much understanding and support from the nursing staff while the nurses gently encourage her to retain as much independence as is compatible with her situation.

Frequently, external and internal radiation therapy is used in conjunction with, or instead of, surgery for these patients. Because a high oxygen concentration in the tissues and blood increases the radiosensitivity of the tumour, anaemia and low circulating blood volumes are corrected before radiation therapy by medication or blood transfusions. Radium in special containers is inserted into the cervical canal and into the lateral fornices of the vagina. The insertion of the radium is an operative procedure. The patient receives a cleansing enema the day before and a perineal shave preparation. During the procedure a urinary catheter with a small balloon is passed. This prevents a distended bladder from coming into contact with the radium, which would greatly increase the chance of a vesicovaginal fistula. After the radium is inserted, packing is placed in the vagina and may be sutured in place to maintain the position of the radium. Because the tight packing prevents the woman emptying her bladder, the catheter drains the bladder. The patient's temperature is monitored, as radiation may stimulate a latent infection. The patient remains on bed-rest with head and shoulders nearly flat. A slipper bedpan is used, and straining at stool is discouraged. The catheter is checked to see that it is draining. These measures help to ensure that the radium remains where it has been placed. Complaints of pain and any bloody discharge should be reported to the doctor. The time for removal should be carefully observed. Removal may be uncomfortable for the patient because of the tight packing, and the patient may need an analgesic for this.

CARCINOMA OF THE ENDOMETRIUM

This is a frequently occurring malignancy which appears to be increasing in incidence. Since it is a disease largely of older women, this may be due to a lengthened life span. Oestrogens aggravate the tumour and prolonged oestrogen therapy, especially in women close to the age of the menopause has been implicated as a contributing cause of endometrial cancer.

The first symptom is a painless, bloody vaginal discharge. Thirty to 40% of women with postmenopausal bleeding have cancer of the endometrium. Bleeding postmenopausally should therefore never be ignored but investigated immediately. A careful endometrial biopsy is usually done. The growth is usually in the fundus of the uterus, but may arise in or spread to the isthmus. The thick body of the uterus contains the growth and it metastasizes late in its growth.

Treatment is by intracavitary radiation followed by a careful total hysterectomy and bilateral salpingo-oophorectomy. Care is taken to pack the vagina or suture the cervix, and tie the tubes to prevent spread by seeding from the uterus. Surgery is often followed by radiation of the vagina as well in order to reduce the risk from stray malignant cells spread during surgery. Some surgeons may do the hysterectomy first and follow with radiation. More advanced cases are treated with combinations of external and internal radiation with surgery to relieve symptoms. Where radium is inserted, several containers attached to strings may be placed in the body of the uterus to irradiate the endometrium. Cure rates are excellent when the tumour has been discovered early.

Progesterone therapy retards the growth of the tumour and metastases. Treatment in the form of medroxyprogesterone acetate (Provera) may be started before surgery and continued for two years afterwards.

CARCINOMA OF THE VAGINA

In recent years there has been an increase in clear cell adenocarcinoma of the vagina in girls and young women. This is a result of *in utero* exposure to diethyl-stilboestrol (DES), a synthetic non-steroid oestrogen compound. DES was first synthesized in 1938; by 1940–41 the drug was prescribed for women to help prevent or treat threatened spontaneous abortion, which was thought to be due to low progesterone levels. Unlike natural oestrogens, it stimulated the body to increase the production of progesterone. The drug was withdrawn from use for this purpose in 1971. Between 1940 and 1971 many thousands of women received treatment with DES. Prior to its withdrawal it had been shown to be a transplacental teratogen and carcinogen, producing a wide range of congenital anomalies of the genital tract in the offspring and a rare vaginal cancer in a few daughters of such pregnancies Table 29.1. During organogenesis, exposure to DES affected Müllerian duct tissue. This tissue remained inappropriately or, in many women, is in the wrong place. Time of exposure was more important than amount of exposure. Disorders following DES exposure *in utero* include physical anomalies, adenosis and carcinoma of the vagina. Estimates vary but 65–95% of at-risk women have cervical and uterine anomalies and about 90% have adenosis. By contrast the risk of

Table 29.1   Effects on girls of exposure to diethylstilboestrol (DES) *in utero*.

1 Congenital anomalies:
   (a) Cervix—hooded, ridged, ringed by fibrous tissue
           —hypoplastic
   (b) Uterus—abnormally shaped, small, internal adhesions, constrictions
   (c) Vagina—transverse ridges
           —stenosis
   (d) Adenosis or ectopic tissue by vagina and cervix
           —this may disappear by age 30
           —not cancer precursor but usually present when cancer occurs
2 Cancer of the genital tract:
   Usually clear cell adenocarcinoma
   Commonest between ages 14–20
   Rare, incidence 1–4 per 1000 at-risk women
3 Increased reproductive difficulties
   Secondary to abnormalities of cervix and uterus
   (a) Primary infertility
   (b) Spontaneous abortion
   (c) Ectopic pregnancy
   (d) Premature labour and delivery

developing cancer is small; perhaps 0.5% of women affected by DES exposure. Although DES induces breast cancer in male mice, there is no evidence at present to indicate that it does so in either sex in humans.

Treatment and nursing care

The regular follow-up and screening visits of those who were exposed to DES begins with the first menstrual period or at age 14 years, whichever is first. Early monitoring of the girl to detect changes at the cellular level involves regular examination every six months including cervical smears, Schiller's test to determine areas of change and hence areas for biopsy, and possibly a colposcopy examination. Cervical smears are only about 75% effective in detecting change in this condition and the cellular screening must be more rigorous and extensive. Women who have not been involved in this early screening programme present with bleeding or a suspicious lesion in the vagina.

Treatment is radical vaginal surgery followed by irradiation and possibly chemotherapy.

Nursing interventions are directed to case-finding by public education and by questioning of appropriate age groups during history taking. Once a case of DES exposure is suspected, teaching about the condition, attendant risks and necessary follow-up is done and the patient is referred to a doctor. The patient and the mother usually require support from professionals and from others in a similar situation.

Adenosis   The signs and symptoms of adenosis include complaints of a heavy clear mucoid discharge, dyspareunia and postcoital bleeding. On inspection, small bright red papillary or granular lesions may be seen on the smooth pink vaginal mucosa. Alternatively, large diffuse red patches may be seen. Numerous small cystic nodules beneath the epithelium are felt on the anterior and posterior vaginal walls. During palpation care must be taken to inspect and palpate the entire vagina as the blades of the speculum may obscure the adenosis. Most adenosis requires no treatment. Extensive adenosis may need cryotherapy or partial vaginectomy with skin grafting.

CARCINOMA OF THE VULVA

Carcinoma of the vulva is a less frequent malignancy, occurring mainly among women in their fifth and sixth decades of life. It is frequently preceded by vulvar changes.

Dystrophy of the vulva

Dystrophy of the vulva refers to changes in vulvar epithelium which are most often associated with ageing but may occur in the younger woman. Most are benign but some are premalignant. Because premalignancy must be assessed at the cellular level a biopsy is done on all lesions.

The patient complains of a shrinking of vulvar structures which progressively narrows the introitus. Dyspareunia, pruritus and soreness are frequent complaints. Smooth red or white patches of thick or thin epithelium may be evident. They may be only in the vestibule or scattered over the vulva and perineum. These patches crack easily, and fissures and excoriated areas develop. Pruritus is common and secondary infection of the scratched lesions occurs. Ulceration may develop.

Mild symptoms usually respond to improved perineal hygiene, control of pruritus and infection and topical application of oestrogen. Patients with more severe symptoms are admitted to the hospital. Nursing care will then involve keeping the vulva dry, cool and clean by daily baths. No pants or pyjamas are worn. The patient is nursed as much as possible with her legs apart and a bed cradle over the perineum to keep it dry and cool. A hair dryer may be used at intervals to blow cool dry air over the perineum. This helps relieve pruritus and promotes healing. It is wise to avoid powders and creams. Medication to reduce the pruritus may be needed as well. If the condition resists treatment or recurs, a simple vulvectomy may be done. Those patients who show signs of cellular changes consistent with an increased risk of developing cancer will have periodical examinations and biopsies done or a simple vulvectomy.

In addition the nurse must observe the vulva and perineum of any patient for whom she cares in order to identify changes which would require further investigation. She should encourage patients who complain of symptoms to her to seek medical attention.

Treatment

Carcinoma of the vulva is treated by radical vulvectomy. Here the dissection is extensive for the clitoris, labia and all the perineal subcutaneous tissue; all the perineal glands and the femoral and inguinal lymphatics are removed.

Nursing care

Preoperative preparation includes all the measures common for perineal and abdominal surgery. The patient and nursing staff may react with repugnance at the thought of this surgery. It is frequently seen as mutilating. However, the results of the operation are quite favourable. Sexual function is retained, as the vagina is not removed. Young women have conceived following simple vulvectomy and have been delivered by caesarean section.

Postoperatively, the patient returns to the ward with an indwelling catheter. Much oedema is present and great care must be taken not to dislodge the catheter. It may be very difficult to replace. The operation may be done in two stages or all at once. In the former, the patient returns with an open area, requiring future skin grafting. Barrier nursing may be required for this patient both before and after skin grafting. A bed cradle over the pubic area will keep bed linen away. When the procedure is completed in one operation the patient may return with a bulky pressure dressing held in place by a T bandage. In other cases there are bilateral stab wounds near the iliac fossa containing drains which are attached to suction; this arrangement may replace the pressure bandage. Thus, the fluid is drained away and the skin flap is kept in close approximation to the underlying tissue so that it becomes firmly attached to the tissue. Some necrosis along the incision lines may be expected, and occasionally skin grafting may be necessary to replace a necrotic area. The stitches are usually not removed for two to three weeks. Close observation is maintained for thromboemboli. Once ambulation is begun, the patient may need elastic stockings to avoid swelling of her legs. Standing for long periods of time should be avoided.

FURTHER READING

Barber, H. R. K. (1980) *Manual of Gynecologic Oncology*. Philadelphia: J. B. Lippincott.

Govan, A. D. *et al*. (1985) *Gynaecology Illustrated*. 3rd edn. Edinburgh: Churchill Livingstone.

Simons, W. (1985) *Learning to Care on the Gynaecology Ward*. Sevenoaks: Hodder & Stoughton.

Smith, P. (1989) New light on lasers. *Nursing Times*, **85** (33) (August 16), 28–31.

TIFFANY, R. (Ed.) (1979) *Cancer Nursing—Radiotherapy*. London: Faber & Faber.

VARMA, T. R. (1986) *Manual of Gynaecology*. Edinburgh: Churchill Livingstone.

WEBB, A. (1989) *Experiences of Hysterectomy*. London: Optima Books.

WELBY-ALLEN, M. (1982) Selectron treatment in gynaecology. *Nursing Times*, (November 17), 1948–1950.

30

DISPLACEMENTS OF THE REPRODUCTIVE TRACT

RETROVERSION AND RETROFLEXION OF THE UTERUS

The normal position of the uterus is one of some anteversion and anteflexion (Fig. 30.1). It is not a fixed organ. The filling of the bladder or bowel may cause a change in uterine position. On occasion, the uterus assumes a retroverted or retroflexed position. When retroverted, the fundus points toward the sacrum and the cervix toward the anterior vaginal wall. Retroflexion refers to the position of the fundus of the uterus in relation to the cervix. In retroflexion the fundus bends back over the cervix (Fig. 30.2). Degrees of retroversion and retroflexion are possible so that the case may be mild or extreme.

The aetiology appears to lie in a weakness of the supporting structures which may be either congenital or acquired. The acquired weakness frequently results from the stresses of pregnancy, labour or delivery. Adhesions and tumours may pull or push the uterus into this position.

The patient may complain of backache, infertility, dyspareunia or dysmenorrhoea, but she is frequently symptomless unless the situation is extreme. Backache and dysmenorrhoea are probably associated with pelvic congestion. Infertility may arise because the cervix does not reach the seminal pool. Frequently, the ovaries prolapse into the cul-de-sac and become

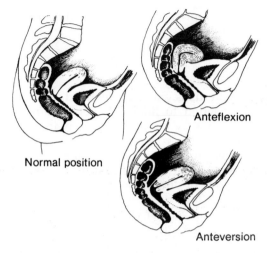

Anteflexion

Normal position

Anteversion

Fig. 30.1 Normal position of the uterus, anteflexion and anteversion.

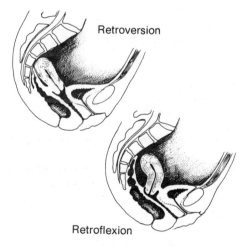

Retroversion

Retroflexion

Fig. 30.2 Retroversion and retroflexion of the uterus.

congested and enlarged. Because of this, intercourse may be painful.

Treatment

Usually the uterus is manually replaced, and a vaginal pessary is inserted to hold the uterus in place. The pessary functions by holding the cervix in a posterior position. This in turn rotates the uterus forward. When the pessary is properly in position, the patient is unaware of its presence and no difficulty is experienced on passing urine or during intercourse. The patient will return in about four to six weeks to have the pessary checked and removed for cleaning. The gynaecologist may then give the patient a six-week trial period without the pessary to see if she remains free of symptoms. If not, a further trial with the pessary may be given.

All pessaries are irritating, especially those which are rubber and have some degree of movement. An offensive-smelling leucorrhoea usually develops, and chronic ulceration may occur.

In other cases the uterus will be surgically suspended by shortening the round ligaments. This is done when the pessary does not correct the situation.

PROLAPSE, CYSTOCELE AND RECTOCELE

Uterine prolapse refers to the downward displacement of the entire organ. Prolapse (Fig. 30.3) may occur in varying degrees. First-degree prolapse describes the condition existing when the uterus descends within the vagina. Second-degree prolapse occurs when the cervix protrudes through the introitus. Procidentia, or third-degree prolapse, refers to the entire uterus protruding through the introitus with total inversion of the vagina.

Cystocele, urethrocele, rectocele and enterocele refer

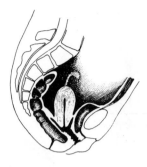

First degree

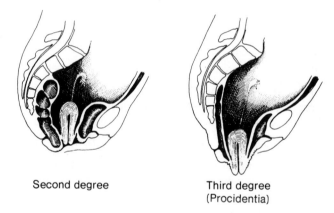

Second degree

Third degree
(Procidentia)

Fig. 30.3 Uterine prolapse, showing first, second and third degree (procidentia) prolapse.

to herniations or relaxations of the bladder, urethra, rectum and small bowel into the vagina (Fig. 30.4). They may occur singly or in combinations with some degree of uterine prolapse.

The single most important aetiological factor in the development of these conditions is thought to be

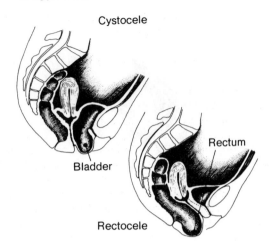

Fig. 30.4   Cystocele and rectocele.

injury at childbirth. The pelvic floor and supporting structures may be stretched and torn during the process of delivery and are thereby weakened. Further relaxation results after menopause as the tissues atrophy following oestrogen withdrawal. Large intra-abdominal tumours may also place an added strain on already weakened tissue. In some rare cases, the structures seem to be congenitally weak.

The patient with a prolapse often complains of a feeling of 'something coming down'. She may have a dragging or a heavy feeling in the pelvis, accompanied by backache and bladder symptoms of either retaining or losing urine. She may have recurrent cystitis. When the cervix protrudes through the introitus, it may become ulcerated from constant friction. This may produce pain and bleeding. The patient with a cystocele frequently has symptoms of stress incontinence.

Diagnosis is usually confirmed by bimanual and rectal examinations. The patient will be asked to bear down, cough or strain while the doctor estimates the degree of prolapse or herniation.

Treatment and nursing responsibilities

The best treatment is prevention. Better care during the pregnancy, labour and the puerperium has helped to reduce the incidence of these complications. Exercises should be taught by the physiotherapist and encouraged by the nurse to all patients in the postpartum period and the same exercises may be taught to help relieve mild prolapse. These consist of alternately tightening and relaxing the gluteal and perineal floor muscles. Practising starting and stopping the stream of urine also helps the patient regain good perineal muscle tone. She should continue to practise these exercises several times a day for several weeks.

In situations in which surgery is contraindicated, the use of pessaries may be employed. A variety are available for different degrees of prolapse.

Surgical intervention is frequently necessary to correct the situation. An anterior and posterior colporrhaphy and perineorrhaphy repair a cystocele and rectocele, respectively.

In some women where prolapse of the uterus is present and future childbearing is not an issue, a Manchester repair may be done. This combines the amputation of an elongated cervix and shortening of the cardinal ligaments with an anterior and posterior repair. Although childbearing is not precluded by an anterior and posterior repair, delivery by caesarean section is usually recommended in order to retain this repair. Vaginal hysterectomy with an anterior and posterior repair is usually performed for more severe uterine prolapse. The uterine tubes and the uterus with all or part of the cervix will be removed. The ligaments and blood vessels are ligated, and a cuff is made in the upper portion of the vagina.

The nursing care of these patients is similar to that given to any patient undergoing surgery. The patient receives a perineal shave preparation. Orders may be given outlining special perineal or vaginal preparations. The nurse assists the patient in understanding the limitations, if any, surgery will impose on sexual and reproductive capacity, since misunderstandings frequently occur.

During surgery the patient may receive an intravenous vasoconstrictor to reduce the danger of haemorrhage. Blood loss during vaginal surgery tends to be heavy and is heavier still in premenopausal women.

The patient's legs are carefully lifted together to be placed into and removed from the stirrups. No one should lean or apply pressure on the anaesthetized leg to avoid thrombus formation. These measures reduce postoperative discomfort, avoid strain on the repaired perineal muscles and help reduce the incidence of postoperative emboli. These same measures should be used whenever a patient's legs are placed in stirrups.

Following vaginal surgery, the nurse observes the patient for signs and symptoms of haemorrhage, urinary tract infection, thromboemboli and infections at the surgical site. Haemorrhage may be frank, oozing or in the form of a large haematoma. The oozing of blood may not be readily noticed by the patient or the staff; therefore, the nurse must be careful to observe the estimated blood loss over a period of time, not just each time she checks the patient. A haematoma is a form of concealed haemorrhage; the blood vessels bleed into the tissue of the vagina or perineum. The patient complains of discomfort or pain over the site. The tissue bulges and may be so taut as to glisten. The nurse should notify the doctor immediately and be prepared to assist with treatment and the possible return of the patient to the operating theatre. Blood transfusions may be required. The clot may be evacuated, the bleeding vessels ligated or the site firmly packed. An antibiotic may be ordered to lessen the chance of infection.

Postoperatively the patient returns with a suprapubic catheter. This is a small polyethylene tube which has been threaded through a needle into the bladder. The abdomen is surgically prepared, the bladder filled with sterile water, and the needle inserted. The tube is taped or caught with a stitch to the skin to avoid accidental removal and attached to a sterile drainage system. It drains freely for three to four days and the patient passes urine as she can. Seventy per cent of women pass urine spontaneously before the tube is clamped, starting on the fourth day. If the tube leaks, tape may be placed around the base. The tube can be used to measure residual urine, but occasionally a catheter may have to be used. Suprapubic drainage has reduced the incidence of postoperative urinary tract infections by reducing the need for urethral catheterizations. They also reduce the emotional tension surrounding first attempts at passing urine.

In some cases the patient may have catheter drainage. She is catheterized preoperatively, and the catheter remains in place for seven to nine days until the oedema has been resolved. The catheter is clamped and released for periods of time, finally removed, and then the patient attempts to pass urine. She is usually catheterized twice daily for residual urine during the first 24–36 hours without the catheter. If the amount of urine remaining in the bladder is above 75–100 ml, a Foley catheter may be reinserted or the cystostomy tube opened.

Voiding in sufficient quantities should occur at least every six hours. To induce the patient who is unable to pass urine to do so requires all the nurse's skill in an attempt to avoid catheterization. Patients are usually encouraged to move about early and getting up to the toilet helps. If the use of a bidet or vulval toilet is allowed, it usually helps if these are encouraged immediately before the patient attempts to pass urine. When catheterization is necessary, the strictest aseptic technique should be followed.

Perineal care is important in the prevention of infection. Depending on the extent of the surgery, sterile technique may be required. It should be as frequent as necessary to keep the perineal area clean and dry. General principles of working from front to back are followed. In addition, sterile pads are applied. Vulval toilet may be ordered with sterile or plain water or some solutions. The nurse or patient runs the solution from a bag and tubing over the perineum into a basin. If the patient is well enough, she is taught how to do these procedures.

Straining at stool is avoided by a low residue diet and the avoidance of constipation.

On discharge the patient may receive further instructions; some doctors definitely restrict heavy lifting and prolonged standing, walking and sitting. Intercourse is contraindicated for approximately six weeks.

FURTHER READING

ANDERSON, A. (1986) *An A–Z of Gynaecology*. London: Faber & Faber. Faber.

GOVAN, A. D. *et al.* (1985) *Gynaecology Illustrated*. 3rd edn. Edinburgh: Churchill Livingstone.

LLEWELLYN-JONES, D. (1972) *Fundamentals of Obstetrics and Gynaecology—Volume 2—Gynaecology*. London: Faber & Faber.

SIMONS, W. (1985) *Learning to Care on the Gynaecology Ward*. Sevenoaks: Hodder and Stoughton.

VARMA, T. R. (1986) *Manual of Gynaecology*. Edinburgh: Churchill Livingstone.

WATSON, J. E. & ROYLE, J. R. (1987) *Watson's Medical-Surgical Nursing and Related Physiology*, 3rd edn. London: Baillière Tindall.

31

COMMON URINARY TRACT PROBLEMS

Because the bladder is closely associated with the genital tract certain urinary problems are common in women. Such problems are particularly common in association with displacement of the uterus.

CYSTITIS

This is one of the commonest complaints with which women consult the general practitioner. It is estimated that perhaps 1.7 million women suffer from cystitis in the UK each year, and of these some may have four to five attacks per year. The problem is often viewed as trivial, but for the woman it is embarrassing and distressing, causing constraints on her life-style.

It is a common complaint when young women become sexually active. It is then thought to be largely due to increased vaginal secretions and vascularity during intercourse and possibly mild trauma caused by the movement of the penis. Because of the close proximity of the anus, vagina and urethra organisms are easily spread; *Escherichia Coli* is a common causative organism of cystitis.

Cystitis may occur as the result of an inflammatory process without bacterial growth and antibiotic treatment will then be unnecessary. The nurse may advise women on ways to help themselves both to reduce the likelihood of attacks and if the problem recurs. In non-bacterial cystitis the urine is acid in reaction and treatment is aimed at restoring an alkaline reaction.

The inflammatory process described may affect the urethra only—the urethral syndrome. This readily ascends to involve the bladder, however.

Causes

Chemical   The use of contraceptive creams, scented soap, 'bubble bath', vaginal deodorants and similar preparations may provoke an attack. Some women are affected after using the swimming pool; others find attacks occur after using a clitoral vibrator.

Some foods such as chillies, pepper or chilli powder, citrus fruit or pickles are irritants for some women. Reduced fluid intake or excessive consumption of coffee or alcohol may precipitate the problem.

Medical   Related problems such as pyelonephritis, renal calculi, urethral stricture, a tumour or foreign body in the bladder, inflammation of the pelvic organs or colon, a cystocele or rectocele may lead to cystitis.

This type of cystitis is likely to have a bacterial cause.

Sexual activity   This is discussed on page 377.

Symptoms

Dysuria—pain and a burning sensation on micturition.
Urgency.
Pain in the lower abdomen and back.
Nausea and sometimes vomiting.
Dark coloured urine which may be offensive; there may be haematuria.
Nocturia.

Preventive self-help

Hygiene measures   Women and girls should always be taught to wipe the vulva and perineum from front to back after using the toilet, and mothers should be similarly advised with baby girls.

If cystitis is related to sexual intercourse the woman should be advised to wash before and after intercourse using plain water. She may like to sit astride the toilet and pour water over the vulval area from a jug.

The use of a detachable shower head is probably safer than soaking in the bath in terms of general hygiene.

No scented soaps or bath preparations should be used.

Clothing   Warm, moist conditions will encourage bacterial growth, so women are advised to wear cotton pants, gussetless tights or stockings, and to avoid wearing tight jeans.

Dietary measures   The woman may be advised to avoid the irritant foods already listed. She should drink plenty of clear fluids every day, and reduce or stop her consumption of tea, coffee, cola drinks and alcohol.

Self-help during an attack

Mid-stream specimen of urine   This should be taken to the doctor as soon as symptoms occur.

Rest   The woman should go to bed and place a covered hot water bottle over the lower abdomen.

Fluid intake   She should aim to drink three to four pints of tap or bottled water containing two teaspoons of bicarbonate of soda over the next few hours.

STRESS INCONTINENCE

Stress incontinence is the involuntary loss of small amounts of urine when a woman coughs, sneezes or otherwise suddenly increases the intra-abdominal pressure and, therefore, the intravesical pressure. It should be distinguished from urge incontinence and frequency.

Continence is thought to be maintained at the junction of the urethra and bladder by continuous spiral muscles from the base of the bladder to the upper urethra. Assistance is also received from the muscles surrounding the urethra, as well as a tight supporting perineal floor. In the continent woman these relationships can be demonstrated radiologically by observing that the angle between the urethra and posterior wall of the bladder is approximately 90° (Fig. 31.1). Normally, this angle is only obliterated at micturition (Fig. 31.2) when an increased intra-abdominal pressure combines with a relaxed urethrovesical muscle and perineal floor to lower the base of the bladder. However, in stress incontinence, the slight effort of straining, coughing or sneezing is sufficient to reduce this angle, and an involuntary loss of urine occurs. This explanation is thought to describe about 90% of cases of stress incontinence. A woman may have a cystocele (Fig. 31.1) and still be continent if the relationships demonstrated by the angle are maintained. However, many women with a cystocele also have accompanying stress incontinence.

Occasionally, stress incontinence follows a cystocele repair. This is probably due to elevation of the bladder to a position which obliterates the angle. For this reason many surgeons check the angle following repair to be sure it will be adequate.

The symptoms may become distressing to the woman. Frequent small dribbles of urine cause wetness, irritation and an offensive odour. The woman

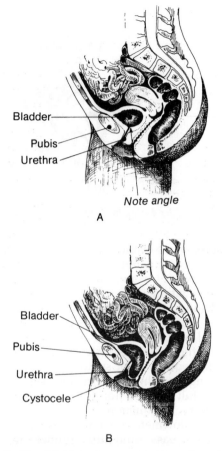

Fig. 31.1 A, The bladder at ease—no stress incontinence, B,
Cystocele without stress incontinence.

may have to wear a perineal pad or plastic pants continuously. Gradually she may become shy of social
contacts and confine herself to home.

Diagnosis is made following a physical examination

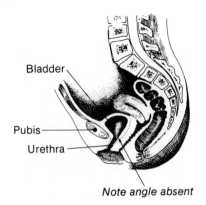

Note angle absent

Fig. 31.2 The bladder during micturition.

and a urodynamic evaluation. A pelvic and modified neurological examination is done to diagnose any underlying pelvic or neurological disease. The uro-dynamic evaluation, which includes a series of tests, helps to distinguish true stress incontinence from other conditions. The series of tests usually requires a day at the hospital and is done on an out-patient basis. In preparation the patient is instructed not to pass urine or take self-medication for six to eight hours if possible before going to the urodynamic laboratory. This provides a full bladder for testing and avoids drug effects on nerve conduction.

Initially uroflowmeter readings are done. The patient is instructed to pass urine into a funnel connected to a flowmeter. This meter is an electronic device which calculates the rate at which urine flows, the time taken to empty the bladder and the volume voided. The results are printed on a graph (Fig. 31.3). An abnormally high rate of flow is associated with stress incontinence. Immediately following this the patient is catheterized for residual urine. This test may be followed by a cystometrogram. During this latter procedure a catheter

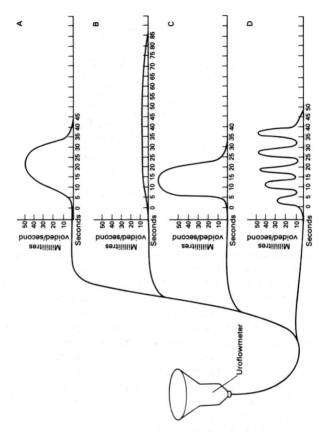

Fig. 31.3 Uroflowmeter flow curves. A, Normal flow pattern; normal rate and peak flow. B, Obstructed flow pattern; long voiding time and low peak. C, Superflow pattern; short voiding time and high peak. D, Abdominal flow pattern; voiding occurs only during periods of increased intra-abdominal pressure (i.e. straining).

is passed, attached to a transducer and the bladder is filled with fluid, usually water. The patient is asked to tell the doctor when she feels a sense of fullness and when her bladder actually feels full. She is told to pass urine and then asked to stop. The transducer meanwhile records on a graph the changes in bladder pressure associated with these events. The doctor can assess how the patient perceives and responds to these sensations and requests. Normally bladder pressure increases during micturition as the bladder is contracting and drops when voiding ceases and the bladder relaxes. This may be combined with a urethral pressure profile. Urethral pressure is recorded as the catheter is slowly withdrawn at a constant rate through the urethra.

More elaborate tests may be done such as electromyograms to measure response and strength of bladder muscle, videorecordings and measurements of intra-abdominal pressure by rectal electrodes. They are used less often in stress incontinence. These tests may be followed by cystourethroscopy in which the urologist directly visualizes the interior of the bladder and urethra. In this procedure a dye outlines the urethra and bladder, demonstrating the state of the angle at rest, during straining and if possible, no micturition.

These procedures, with the exception of the uroflowmeter, require sterile equipment, appropriate preparation of the patient and sterile gowning and gloving of the staff. A few patients may require an anaesthetic.

Treatment

Treatment begins with prevention of injury and ensuing incontinence by good maternity care and the practice of postpartum exercises in the immediate postpartum period.

Stress incontinence is aggravated by chronic urinary

tract infections, obesity and chronic coughing. Prevention includes the education of women about stress
incontinence and the aggravating factors. Any urinary
and vaginal tract infections are treated; the obese
patient is advised to lose weight and an appropriate
diet is discussed to assist her with this. The heavy
smoker is advised to reduce or stop smoking as a
means of reducing coughing, and is also instructed
about stop-smoking programmes designed to help in
this. The patient is assisted to re-establish a normal
pattern of micturition and bladder control. She is
usually provided with a bladder drill and exercise
regimen.

Bladder drill involves routines related to micturition.
The patient is instructed to pass urine each hour by the
clock whether she feels the need to or not. When she
has kept herself dry this way for three or four days she
increases the time interval between voidings by one-
half hour every three days until she can comfortably
hold urine for three hours. She is instructed to drink
plenty of non-stimulating fluids (e.g. caffeine-free)
during the day, to drink nothing for two hours before
going to bed and to empty her bladder completely
before going to sleep. She is also instructed to empty
her bladder before and after sexual intercourse.

The exercises consist of always giving an extra push
at the end of micturition to make sure all urine is
expelled. She also is instructed to practise tightening
the buttocks and pelvic floor muscles and stopping and
starting the stream of urine during micturition. The
exercises are practised several times a day. If the
patient is unsure whether or not she is practising them
correctly, she can be taught to insert two fingers into
the vagina and contract the vaginal muscles to grip the
fingers as tightly as possible. This provides the patient
with a direct measure of her progress. Once she has
learned the technique, it can be practised without
inserting her fingers.

Various smooth muscle relaxants which inhibit detrusor activity and increase bladder capacity may be prescribed while the patient is practising the bladder drill and re-establishing a good pattern.

If this regimen is unsuccessful, and in cases of prolapse with urethral incompetence, surgery may be necessary in order to support the urethra and restore the proper urethrovesical relationship.

Two types of operations are commonly used. In the Aldridge sling operation the surgeon makes a sling of fascia. This sling is then attached to the anterior abdominal wall. This serves to support the urethra, which can be demonstrated by observing the restoration of the angle. The approach may be abdominal, vaginal or both. Occasionally, the sling is too tight and the patient has difficulty micturating and emptying the bladder properly. Cystitis and other complications may occur. Teaching the patient to bend her body forward when attempting to void postoperatively helps. This relaxes the muscles of the abdomen, thereby loosening the sling and lowering the base of the bladder.

The Marshall–Marchetti–Krantz operation supports the urethra by suturing the anterior vaginal wall on each side to the periosteum of the pubic bone and the anterior wall of the bladder to the pubic bone.

The two most common operations performed in the UK are the Burch colposuspension (which has an estimated 85% success rate) and the anterior vaginal repair operation (with an estimated 30% success rate).

In the Burch colposuspension operation the procedure is carried out abdominally. The vagina is lifted by means of two sutures inserted into each side of the bladder and then attached to the iliopectoral ligament.

Urinary tract problems associated with pregnancy are discussed in Chapters 9 and 10.

FURTHER READING

GOULD, D. (1990) *Nursing Care of Women.* Englewood Cliffs, NJ: Prentice-Hall.

SHREARE, C. (1986) *Cystitis—the New Approach.* Wellingborough: Thorsons.

WATSON, J. E. & ROYLE, J. R. (1987) *Watson's Medical-Surgical Nursing and Related Physiology,* 3rd edn. London: Baillière Tindall.

32

THE BREASTS AND ASSOCIATED PROBLEMS

Problems associated with the postnatal period and lactation are discussed in Chapter 17.

The breasts are an obvious indication of femininity. Women tend to be very conscious of their size and shape and are frequently dissatisfied with these. In Western society the breasts are very much associated with sexual attractiveness whereas for some women in other cultures they may be purely utilitarian—for feeding infants.

For Western women, then, any breast problem may pose a threat to sexual attractiveness, body image and self-acceptance. Such a threat may be real or imagined. Not every problem will require surgery, but breast surgery will be felt as mutilating and may cause great distress and anguish.

ASSESSMENT

History

A detailed history is taken of the individual's: (1) age; (2) health history; (3) family history of illness and disorders of the breasts; (4) parity and nursing of infant(s); (5) menstrual history (age of onset, regularity, menopause); (6) date of discovery of lesion; (7) symptoms (detailed description) that prompted patient's visit to the doctor; (8) knowledge of risk factors associated with breast cancer; (9) breast self-examination practices; and (10) feelings concerning the meaning of the breast to the individual's femininity.

Physical examination of the breasts

Inspection With the patient uncovered to the waist, the breasts are observed with the patient sitting upright, leaning forward and lying down.

Palpation The breasts are then palpated with the patient in the supine and sitting position. The entire breast is examined in a systematic manner, beginning in one quadrant and moving around until the starting point is again reached. The normal breast varies in consistency and may feel granular in older individuals. If any masses are discovered they are palpated for size, shape, consistency, mobility, discreteness of borders, location and tenderness. The infraclavicular, cervical and axillary areas are palpated for enlarged lymph nodes.

Diagnostic tests

Prompt, thorough medical investigation is indicated when any changes or symptoms are observed.

Mammogram This is an X-ray procedure used in breast examination without the injection of a contrast medium. A series of X-rays of the breasts is made from two planes, from above and lateral. The films are examined for any areas of increased density and, if present, their characteristics (location, size, shape, regularity of borders). A lesion may be detected in a mammogram before it becomes palpable.

Xerograph Xerography involves the use of an aluminium plate with an electrically charged coat of selenium. On X-ray exposure, an electrostatic image is transferred to paper by a special process. The xerogram provides more accurate, detailed information about the soft tissues of the breast than the mammogram.

Thermogram   The skin over some tumours of the breast is warmer than that over normal areas. A thermogram may be made of the breast with an infrared camera to detect these areas of higher temperature.

Biopsy   Biopsy provides a specimen of tissue for cytological examination; the specimen may be obtained by aspiration, resection or excision. In the case of breast tumours, most surgeons prefer an excision biopsy, since it permits an examination of the complete tumour.

Bone scans   In patients with malignant tumours of the breast, especially when axillary lymph node involvement is identified, bone scans are done to identify bone metastases.

Manifestations of breast disorders

Symptoms of breast disorders may be insidious and may include: alterations in the size and/or shape of the breasts; palpable masses in the breast tissue and discharge from the nipples. The size and shape of breasts vary among individual females and with age. Very large breasts may cause physical discomfort by the weight they impose on shoulders and other parts. Attitudes towards breast size are individual and are greatly influenced by social values, clothing styles and the person's self-image and femininity. Changes in the symmetry of the breasts may be caused by pathological processes. Palpable masses in the breasts may not be tender but are frequently discovered by women during self-examination of their breasts.

Breast self-examination

Regular self-examination of the breasts plays an important role in early detection of a breast lesion.

Breast cancer is the most common malignancy in women, accounting for approximately 26% of newly diagnosed carcinomas in females each year.

Many women do not examine their breasts routinely. All women from their early teens onward should be taught to examine their breasts monthly and to see a doctor promptly if any changes are observed.

Every nurse has the responsibility, as well as frequent opportunity, to teach patients and friends the importance and procedure of regular self-examination of the breasts. It should not be assumed that women have been taught the procedure or that they perform self-examination of the breasts thoroughly and routinely.

A variety of resources, including leaflets films and videos, are availabe for teaching breast self-examination.

The importance of monthly breast self-examination

Women should be aware that 90% of breast tumours are initially identified by women themselves. A high percentage of breast carcinomas are palpable and can be detected early at a size of about 1 cm. Routine breast examination increases the likelihood of early detection and thus improved prognosis, as the chance of metastasis is decreased in the early stages of the disease.

Risk factors   Breast cancer is more likely to occur to women who: are older (the incidence increases sharply with age until menopause and again five years postmenopause); live in North America or northern Europe; have fibrocystic disease of the breast; have no children, or have their first child after the age of 30 years; have a family history of breast cancer; are Jewish; and have an early menarche or a late menopause, or both.

In the shower:

Examine your breasts during bath or shower; hands glide easier over wet skin. Fingers flat, move gently over every part of each breast. Use right hand to examine left breast, left hand for right breast. Check for any lump, hard knot or thickening.

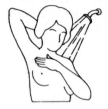

Before a mirror:

Inspect your breasts with arms at your sides. Next, raise your arms high overhead. Look for any changes in contour of each breast,

a swelling, dimpling of skin or changes in the nipple.

Then, rest palms on hips and press down firmly to flex your chest muscles. Left and right breast will not exactly match—few women's breasts do.

Regular inspection shows what is normal for you and will give you confidence in your examination.

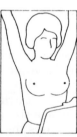

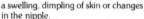

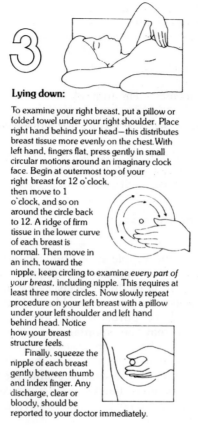

Lying down:

To examine your right breast, put a pillow or folded towel under your right shoulder. Place right hand behind your head — this distributes breast tissue more evenly on the chest. With left hand, fingers flat, press gently in small circular motions around an imaginary clock face. Begin at outermost top of your right breast for 12 o'clock, then move to 1 o'clock, and so on around the circle back to 12. A ridge of firm tissue in the lower curve of each breast is normal. Then move in an inch, toward the nipple, keep circling to examine *every part of your breast*, including nipple. This requires at least three more circles. Now slowly repeat procedure on your left breast with a pillow under your left shoulder and left hand behind head. Notice how your breast structure feels.

Finally, squeeze the nipple of each breast gently between thumb and index finger. Any discharge, clear or bloody, should be reported to your doctor immediately.

Fig. 32.1 Self-examination of the breast—an example of a teaching leaflet.

Risk factors are assessed in relation to the individual and are re-evaluated with age and changes in health status.

Self-examination of the breast The examination should be made regularly each month, a few days after menstruation, and should be continued after menopause. It involves inspection before a mirror and palpation while bathing and then in the supine position. See Fig. 32.1 for a description and diagram of the techniques of breast self-examination.

Expected outcomes   The individual:

1. Is able to list risk factors for breast cancer that apply to her.
2. Demonstrates the technique of breast self-examination on herself and/or a model.
3. Performs breast self-examination every month.

DISORDERS OF THE NIPPLE

Drainage from the nipple in a non-lactating breast is usually a result of an intraductal papilloma, carcinoma, mammary dysplasia or ductal ectasia (distension). The discharge is usually serous or bloody but may be milky, brownish or purulent and may be unilateral or bilateral. It may be spontaneous or occur with manipulation. The breasts are assessed for a mass, and a history is taken to determine whether there is any relationship between the drainage and menstruation and if the patient is taking oral contraceptives or oestrogen therapy for postmenopausal symptoms.

BENIGN TUMOURS OF THE BREAST

Fibrocystic disease and benign epithelial hyperplasia

These are relatively common disorders of the female breast and are characterized predominantly by fibroplasia, epithelial hyperplasia and the formation of cysts. The lesions are influenced by a hormonal imbalance, are usually bilateral and occur most often in women 30–50 years of age, with a higher incidence in those approaching menopause. A painless mass is usually the first and only manifestation; occasionally there may be some tenderness. The patient may experience more severe soreness and pain of the breasts than is usual in the premenstrual period.

The cysts may be aspirated under local anaesthesia. If a solid mass is encountered or the aspirated fluid contains blood, an incisional biopsy may be performed to rule out carcinoma. Following the initial aspiration, the patient is re-examined periodically and aspiration of recurrent or newly formed cysts may be necessary. Fibrocystic disease is believed to increase the risk of breast cancer. The disease regresses with the onset of menopause.

Fibroadenoma

Fibroadenoma is a benign tumour which develops most frequently in young women. It generally occurs singly, but rarely there may be more than one. Although it is not usually encapsulated, it remains localized and is freely movable and usually painless. Medical authors indicate no increased tendency to subsequent carcinoma in patients who have had a fibroadenoma.

The treatment consists of local excision of the tumour, which is submitted for cytological examination for confirmation of the diagnosis of nonmalignancy.

Patients admitted for biopsy and confirmatory diagnosis of a benign breast growth have very specific nursing needs related to their diagnosis.

The potential problems of these patients include:

1. Failure to adjust to the diagnosis and to accept that the lump is benign.

2. Inability to appreciate the need for regular breast self-examination.

3. Non-acceptance of the results of treatment (or non-treatment—for example scarring, disfigurement and discomfort).

Patients who are offered surgical removal of the growth are potentially at risk of developing many of the problems associated with surgery of malignant growths, especially those concerning self-image and the development of appropriate coping mechanisms.

Nursing intervention

Nursing intervention for patients with *benign* breast disorders includes assessment of the patient's emotional responses to the disorder and biopsy, instruction regarding breast self-examination and measures to reduce the physical symptoms.

The emotional response of individuals to the diagnosis of a benign breast tumour or scarring and possible disfigurement from a biopsy varies with the individual and the degree of the perceived threat to her self-image and femininity. The nurse assesses the patient's response and allows opportunity for the patient to express her feelings and concerns. A referral may be made to the general practitioner and a community nurse.

Breast self-examination is taught to all patients and the importance of regular, monthly examination is stressed.

Measures which may help alleviate the physical symptoms of the disorder are explained if relevant to the individual. Such measures include: (1) wearing a brassière 24 hours a day to provide firm support for the breast and to ease discomfort associated with movement; (2) use of heat or cold applications or mild analgesics to relieve discomfort; and (3) altering diet to eliminate caffeine, theophylline and theobromine.

CARCINOMA

The breast is the most common site of cancer in the female. It rarely occurs under the age of 25, and the incidence progressively increases with age. The greatest number of patients develop their disease between the ages of 40 and 50.

The cause of breast cancer is unknown. Three factors presently being considered are: (1) hormonal, (2) viral, and (3) genetic.

Many malignant tumours of the breast appear to be influenced by ovarian hormones, especially oestrogen. It has been demonstrated that some patients with cancer of the breast have a remission of their disease when the oestrogen concentration is reduced by oophorectomy, adrenalectomy, hypophysectomy or by the administration of anti-oestrogenic agents.

Age, hereditary predisposition and a prior history of breast cancer are the most significant factors influencing the risk of developing breast cancer.

Signs and symptoms

The earliest symptom is generally a single, painless, non-tender mass which is poorly circumscribed and may have a nodular surface. It is usually discovered by the patient when bathing or during a routine self-examination of the breasts. Other symptoms which may develop include change in the size or contour of the affected breast, retraction of the nipple or an area of the skin over the breast, bleeding or discharge from the nipple, a scaly rash around the nipple, enlargement of axillary or infra- or supraclavicular lymph nodes or a bleeding, ulcerated area on the breast surface.

As the cancer grows, it spreads to adjacent tissues, such as the skin and underlying fascia and muscle. Retraction is due to involvement of the supporting fibrous tissue; there is a proliferation of fibroblasts and ensuing scar tissue within the breast and fascia of the chest muscles. The breast becomes firmer and cannot be moved as freely. Ulceration is associated with advanced disease which has spread to involve the skin.

Metastases

Cancer of the breast may spread directly into adjacent structures or may metastasize to distant structures by emboli of tumour cells being transported through the lymphatics or the blood vessels. The axillary, supra-clavicular or mediastinal lymph nodes are usually the first site of secondary involvement. Other structures which frequently become the site of metastases are the lungs, liver, spine, pelvic bones and femora.

Records show that progress relative to cure and survival of persons with cancer of the breast has been disappointing. It is suggested that a majority of the women have metastasis at the time of diagnosis and primary treatment.

Surgical treatment

Radical mastectomy is the operation adopted by many surgeons and involves removal of the complete breast, the underlying pectoralis (major and minor) muscles and the axillary lymphatics and lymph nodes. A large area of the overlying skin is removed and, if the remaining skin flaps cannot be approximated without a good deal of tension, a skin graft is done. The anterior surface of the thigh is the usual donor site.

A *modified radical mastectomy* is a more conservative procedure which removes the breast, axillary lymphatics and lymph nodes and leaves the pectoral muscles. This is frequently the operation performed when the patient's disease is found to be in the earlier stages. Removal of the breast leaving the axillary lymphatics, lymph nodes and pectoral muscles intact comprises a *simple mastectomy*.

A *lumpectomy* involves removal of the tumour, leaving the breast intact.

Radiation implantation

As early as 1924 surgeons were attempting to treat breast cancer with local implantation, but until recently results were vastly better using external beam treatment. In recent clinical trials patients had local tumour removal leaving the breast intact, removal of the draining lymph nodes, whole breast and lymph node irradiation and direct radiation using interstitial implants of iridium-192 to the tumour site, with marked improvement in results.

Radiation therapy

External radiation therapy may be used as an adjunct to surgery or alone in cases in which the disease is advanced and inoperable, or in which there is a local recurrence after surgery.

Chemotherapy

There is an increasing use of chemotherapeutic agents as an adjunct to mastectomy in the treatment of breast cancer. Combinations of anticancer drugs are usually used.

Adjuvant chemotherapy is prescribed over a long term—one or more years. The drugs are circulated in the blood throughout the body, reaching areas of metastatic disease. They are toxic to many normal cells in addition to cancerous cells, and have severe side-effects.

Hormone deprivation

As cited earlier, some patients with carcinoma of the breast experience a remission of their disease when the concentration of certain hormones (mainly oestrogen) is reduced. Their cancer is said to be hormone-dependent. Cells in some breast cancers have a high affinity for oestrogen; these cells are referred to as oestrogen-receptor cells.

The patient may have an oophorectomy (removal of the ovaries), especially if she is premenopausal. This reduces the production of both oestrogen and pro-gesterone. An adrenalectomy or hypophysectomy may also be done to decrease the production of oestrogen if the patient has shown a favourable response to an oophorectomy. The patient who has an adrenalectomy will require cortisone replacement therapy. If a com-plete hypophysectomy is done, the administration of cortisone and thyroid extract will be necessary because of the removal of the respective tropic hormones (ACTH and TSH), as well as a vasopressin (Pitressin) pre-paration to replace the antidiuretic hormone (ADH).

The administration of an androgen (male hormone) may be prescribed alone or in conjunction with one of the above surgical procedures.

Preoperative care

Women about to undergo mastectomy will usually experience anticipatory grieving related to the loss of a breast, potential threat to life, potential disfigurement and the potential or actual diagnosis of cancer and alteration in body image and femininity.

Nursing intervention

Giving information   The goal is to help the patient understand the hospital routines, the surgical procedure and pre- and postoperative care.

The nurse explains hospital routines and procedures to the patient and family and, if possible, introduces them to a member of the nursing staff of the operating theatre.

Deep breathing, coughing and arm exercises are demonstrated by the nurse and opportunity is provided for the patient to practise them.

The patient is informed that fluids will be administered intravenously postoperatively, what measures will be provided to relieve pain and how the nurse will assist her with deep breathing and coughing and in performing arm exercises. The type of drainage system to be used in the incision is also described.

The nurse assesses the patient's understanding of the diagnosis and operative procedure, reinforces information provided by the surgeon and allows the patient and family to ask questions, express concerns and explore the implications of the surgery for them.

If there has not been a previous biopsy to determine if the mass is benign or malignant, the patient may be uncertain of the extent of surgery to be performed. Before operation, the surgeon explains to the patient and the family the procedure that will be followed and the operative consent form indicates 'biopsy and possible radical mastectomy'.

The patient must be informed of the possibility and must sign the consent form for a mastectomy, or the mastectomy will be performed at a later date following the biopsy. The patient is then able to make an informed decision about the extent of the surgery to be performed.

Anticipatory grieving   The goals are to:

1. Reduce anxiety and fear.
2. Express feelings and concerns.

The general public has become more aware of cancer but, unfortunately, many people do not realize that a large number of cancer patients who receive early treatment are cured. To many, the word cancer only implies suffering, mutilation and death. In many instances fear of learning the truth leads to delay in seeking medical advice.

The impact of being advised of the need for a biopsy and possible radical mastectomy if the mass is cancerous understandably evokes fears and emotional reactions in the patient. Her anxiety may be focused upon suffering, disfigurement, loss of femininity, or death. How she will react is unpredictable; responses and behaviour vary depending on background and previous experiences. One patient may appear quite unconcerned but actually is in turmoil underneath her composure. Some may be withdrawn and unresponsive, others are angry and resentful that this should happen to them, and a few may be actually disorganized. The patient may have feelings of helplessness, loneliness and abandonment. Each patient requires the support of a nurse who understands and appreciates what the implications of the situation may be for the woman and her family.

Physical preparation Usually, there is a minimal period of preparation; the surgery is considered urgent in order to prevent spread of the disease if possible. Investigation to detect metastases may include a chest X-ray, liver and bone scanning and determination of the alkaline phosphatase concentration in the blood. The patient's blood is typed and cross-matched, and blood is made available for transfusion. Her general condition is assessed, and full blood count and haemoglobin estimations are made. If anaemia is present, a transfusion may be ordered preoperatively. The fluid intake is increased to ensure optimum hydration.

The local skin preparation (shaving and cleansing) is ordered by the surgeon. It usually extends from above the clavicle to the umbilical level, and from the nipple line on the unaffected side to the back on the affected side, and includes the axilla and the arm to the elbow. If the surgeon anticipates the need for skin grafting, preparation of an indicated donor site will be necessary. A sedative is generally given the night before operation to ensure adequate rest.

Postoperative care following lumpectomy

If the patient's surgery involves only resection of a tumour and not mastectomy, nursing intervention related to the patient's physiological needs is minimal. A nurse remains with the patient until she recovers from the anaesthetic; she is then made comfortable and is left to rest. The doctor visits to advise her of the pathological findings. She may be permitted to be up later that day or the next morning and, if no further surgery is required, she is usually discharged from the hospital on the second or third postoperative day. The sutures are removed in five to seven days.

Postoperative care following mastectomy

Potential patient problems

1. Potential for injury and complications due to surgical intervention and incomplete healing process.
2. Alteration in comfort: acute pain related to surgical intervention and anxiety.
3. Ineffective breathing pattern related to surgical intervention, pain and discomfort.
4. Alteration in nutrition: less than body require-

ments, related to decreased oral intake following surgery and anaesthesia, and increased body needs for repair and healing.

5. Ineffective individual coping mechanisms, related to loss of a breast, the threat of death and altered self-image.

6. Impaired mobility, pain, discomfort and oedema of the affected arm related to the surgical procedure.

7. Disturbance in self-image related to loss of breast.

8. Lack of knowledge about wound care, protection and use of the affected arm and follow-up health care.

1. Potential for injury and complications   The goals are to:

1. Maintain body functioning.
2. Prevent complications.
3. Promote healing.

Assessment   The breast has an abundant blood supply, which increases the blood loss during surgery and the risk of postoperative haemorrhage. Close observation of the patient is maintained during the first 36–48 hours to detect early signs of shock or haemorrhage. The dressings are inspected for blood, and the bedding under the affected side is also checked, the space between the chest wall and the skin may be drained by a tube brought out through a stab wound and attached to a wound suction receptacle (Redivac). The amount and colour of the drainage are noted at frequent intervals, and any indication of bleeding is reported at once.

The patient's blood pressure, pulse, colour and responses are recorded at frequent intervals. Her reaction to the mastectomy is also noted, since emotional disturbance may contribute to shock. Throughout the patient's hospitalization, the affected arm is checked frequently for oedema and, after 48 hours, the range of motion.

Positioning When the patient is responding fully, the head of the bed is gradually elevated to promote wound drainage. The patient is turned on the unaffected side every two hours. The affected arm is immobilized for 24 hours to prevent haemorrhage and wound strain. The hand is raised so that it is higher than the elbow. When moving or turning the patient, the arm is *gently* lifted, and any abduction and extension that might increase wound tension are avoided. Arm exercises are started early in the postoperative period, beginning with movements of the hand, wrist and elbow.

Wound care The dressing is quite bulky and, unless there is bleeding, is usually left undisturbed for several days. The drainage tube may be removed on the second or third day, depending on the amount of drainage. Sutures are removed in seven to nine days; the surgeon may request the removal of alternate sutures, leaving the remainder for a few days longer. If a skin graft has been done, the donor site dressing may be removed in three to four days, leaving the area exposed.

2. Alteration in comfort The goal is to control pain and discomfort.

An analgesic such as morphine or pethidine is prescribed for the relief of pain during the first 48 hours. A milder analgesic such as codeine is then used if necessary. Turning the patient, slightly changing her position and alternate flexion and extension of the fingers and hand and forearm of the affected arm to promote relaxation or adjustment of supporting pillows may also contribute to the relief of discomfort.

3. Ineffective breathing pattern The goal is to maintain respiratory functioning.

The respirations are likely to be shallow because of

the chest wound. To prevent pulmonary complications, the patient is encouraged to take several deep breaths and cough at frequent intervals during the first few days postoperatively. Gentle support to the affected side while deep breathing and coughing may lessen the discomfort and be reassuring to the patient.

4. Alteration in nutrition   The goal is to maintain nutritional and fluid status.

There is a considerable loss of blood and fluid during a radical mastectomy. A blood transfusion is frequently given during the surgery or immediately afterwards. Fluids are given intravenously throughout the day of operation to replace the loss and may be continued until sufficient quantities are taken orally. The patient is given fluids by mouth as soon as she can tolerate them and is progressed to a regular diet accordingly.

5. Ineffective individual coping mechanism   The goals are to:

1. Reduce emotional distress.
2. Develop constructive coping skills.

The patient who has had a mastectomy requires a great deal of support and needs to know that someone understands her problems. The psychological impact of having cancer and experiencing the loss of a breast is great and, even though the patient was well prepared before operation, shock and depression follow, especially when the dressing is removed and the operative area is seen. The nurse indicates a willingness to listen to the patient, acknowledging and accepting her reactions. If she is withdrawn, she is encouraged to talk and express her despair.

Denial (part of the grieving process) and other coping mechanisms break down over time and awareness of the loss increases. Most women cope effectively with the experience within three months to a year following surgery.

Long-term support for the patient is necessary; identification of people who the patient feels can provide support throughout hospitalization and recovery is important.

Friends provide additional support for the patient, as do women who have had a mastectomy. The patient is informed of community health services available to her, The Mastectomy Association and local self-help groups such as 'Coping with Cancer' and BACUP. These groups enable patients to give and receive support as well as to share experiences.

It is helpful to talk with the family, especially the partner, to alert them to the patient's depression and fear of rejection and to seek their cooperation. The family should tactfully show that their relationships have not changed and that the patient is still acceptable to them. The partner is advised of the marked change in physical appearance and told that this can be corrected by prosthesis.

6. Impaired mobility of the affected arm   The goal is to restore normal functioning of the affected arm.

The patient is usually assisted out of bed the day after the operation if her vital signs are stable. The affected arm is supported to decrease tension, oedema and discomfort caused by movement and dependency. A nurse remains with her to determine her reaction and provides support when she is walking or going to the toilet because her balance and accustomed pattern of movement are interfered with by the immobilization of the arm.

Exercise of the affected arm is necessary soon after the operation to promote circulation and lymph drainage, prevent contracture and limited range of movement and restore normal function.

The initial exercises are begun slowly; the frequency,

vigour and range of movement are progressively increased from day to day according to the woman's tolerance. Using the affected arm in the performance of self-care activities such as washing the face, bathing, cleaning the teeth and brushing and combing the hair is encouraged by the nurse.

A more formalized programme of exercises is planned and started for the individual patient or for a group of patients in hospital at the same time by the physiotherapist. These generally include pulley motion, rope-turning, pendulum-swinging, climbing the wall with the hands, and rod raising. Additional exercises may be included later.

The Mastectomy Association (24 Harrison Street, King's Cross, London WC1) have a booklet which illustrates and gives directions for postmastectomy exercises and activities as well as useful information on prostheses. A supply of these booklets should be kept available on the surgical ward for use in teaching the patient exercises. A copy is also given to the patient.

Oedema of the arm   The removal of axillary lymphatics and lymph nodes in radical mastectomy predisposes to oedema and swelling of the arm after operation.

7. Disturbance in self-image   The goals are to:

1. Identify impact of disease and surgery on body image and sexuality.
2. Restore feelings of attractiveness.
3. Discuss ways of maintaining sexual identity.

Reintegration of body image following mastectomy occurs gradually. Supporting the woman in looking at, feeling and touching the incision helps her to become aware of, and acknowledge, the change in her appearance.

The patient is encouraged to be fitted for a brassière

with a prosthesis. Prosthesis manufacturers have brochures that should be kept available for exploration by the patient. The nurse shows the patient how to pad the brassières she has with absorbent cotton covered with soft cotton so they can be used until a properly fitted prosthesis can be worn. The surgeon will indicate when the wound is sufficiently healed that she may wear a prosthesis. The nurse can provide information, foster open communication between the patient and spouse and encourage them to discuss ways of expressing sexuality and maintaining sexual identity. Breast reconstruction may be possible and should be discussed with the surgeon.

If the wound is not completely healed and requires cleansing and dressing, the patient or a member of her family is taught the necessary procedure, or a referral may be made to the district nurse.

8. Lack of knowledge The goals are to help the patient to:

1. Understand the treatment plan, wound care, arm protection and exercises and availability of community resources.

2. Develop a plan for continuing care and therapy.

The patient is advised that extra precautions should be taken to protect the arm on the operative side. This is necessary because of the loss of the defence mechanisms (lymph nodes, and the lowered resistance associated with the disease), irradiation and chemotherapy. Cuts, scratches, burns and constrictions (e.g. blood pressure cuff or watch with elastic strap) should be avoided. The arm is protected by carrying the handbag and heavy articles on the other arm. The arm should not be used for the withdrawal of blood specimens or receiving injections. Jewellery (watch, bracelet, rings) should be worn loosely in case the arm or hand becomes oedematous, resulting in constriction and difficulty in removing rings or a bracelet. The identification card carried by the individual should indicate that needle injections and constriction should not be used on the affected arm, and why (mastectomy lymphoedema). A 'Medic Alert' pendant or bracelet may be obtained that indicates the need for caution.

If a series of radiation treatments or chemotherapy is to be given, the surgeon discusses this with the patient and advises her when the treatment will commence. It is not usually instituted until the wound is healed, and it may be given on an out-patient basis. The doctor also informs the patient as to when she may resume her household activities or return to her former occupation. The resumption of former activities is encouraged just as soon as the patient is well enough. It relieves her depression and leaves her less time to concentrate on her disease. Use of the involved arm is encouraged and arm exercises should be carried out daily as scheduled.

A close follow-up is necessary; the patient is required to make frequent visits to her doctor or the cancer clinic during the first year or two. Then, if there has been no evidence of recurrence of her disease, the interval between examinations is lengthened to six months or one year.

All patients are taught self-examination of the breast and are informed of the importance of examining the remaining breast each month.

A series of tests including liver and bone scans and blood tests are performed to rule out the presence of metastasis.

Once chemotherapy has begun, the patient requires information about the actions and side-effects of the drugs and measures that help prevent or alleviate adverse reactions. If the patient experiences nausea, an anti-emetic is given with each treatment. Fluid intake is increased to prevent bladder irritation from cyclo-phosphamide. Relaxation techniques may be taught to decrease the nausea following treatment. The nurse helps the patient establish a schedule for medication that is least disruptive to her life-style. For example, medications may be given on Friday afternoons for women who are working, allowing her to remain at home over the weekend when adverse effects from the drugs are most likely to occur.

MAMMOPLASTY

Mammoplasty is surgical intervention to alter the size and shape of the breasts. *Augmentation mammoplasty* is done to enlarge the breasts and involves the placement of a Silastic prosthesis in a surgically constructed pocket between the capsule of the breast and the pectoral fascia.

Breast reduction involves removal of breast tissue to construct breasts that are more normal in size and shape.

The breast holds significance for all women and has a profound impact on self-image and sexuality. Breasts that are too small or too large by cultural or individual standards do affect how the individual views herself and how she relates to others. Rationale for the surgery is very individualistic.

Large breast reduction surgery is also done to relieve backache and shoulder pain. Large breasts may also interfere with activities such as driving a car, or operating machines. They can be equally as embarrassing to the individual as small breasts.

Breast reconstruction may be done following mastectomy. Newer techniques enable the creation of a breast that resembles the natural breast in size, shape and feel. The patient's nipple may be implanted in the inguinal area at the time of the mastectomy and later used in the breast reconstruction.

FURTHER READING

CAHOON, M. C. (Ed.) (1982) *Cancer Nursing*, Chapter 3. Edinburgh: Churchill Livingstone.

MARKS-MARAN, D. & POPE, B. M. (1985) *Breast Cancer Nursing and Counselling*. Oxford: Blackwell Scientific Publications.

MCPHERSON, A. & ANDERSON, A. (1983) *Women's Problems in General Practice*. Oxford University Press.

STANWAY, A. & STANWAY, P. (1982) *The Breast*. Granada.

WATSON, J. E. & ROYLE, J. R. (1987) *Watson's Medical-Surgical Nursing and Related Physiology*, 3rd edn. London: Baillière Tindall.

33

WOMEN AND HEALTH ISSUES

As medical knowledge advances and more diseases can be detected and cured, so demands on the health service of any country will increase in proportion. Even the richest country has finite resources, however, and the provisions made will always have a political implication.

Just as women have gradually become less subservient, more assertive and more vocal during the twentieth century, they have become more aware of their health and that of their families, and have become more confident in seeking health care. This is not yet true throughout the entire population. Women in the lower socio-economic groups remain underprivileged and at greater risk of health problems, yet are less able and willing to seek or even accept help for themselves.

Women face many pressures and conflicts during adult life. Many are attempting to bring up a family and pursue a career; others have small children but are struggling with a reduced income because they do not work for pay outside the home, or have the pressures of being a lone parent. Society presents a variety of conflicting messages to women. These include the message that motherhood is an attractive, rewarding occupation, that success in a career is good, that children are best cared for by their mothers, that child-care is a mundane occupation.

Advertising presents the ideal home, always clean, tidy and hygienic, full of the latest gadgets and fashion-

ably decorated; such perfection is achieved by means
of easily obtained credit is the message. Imagine the
feelings of the young mother who is struggling alone
in her high-rise council flat or temporary accommo-
dation with too little money to feed her family with
healthy food, or with the shadow of accumulating
debts hanging over her.

Small children are exhausting and demanding as
well as rewarding, and many mothers may be more
aware of the former than the latter, especially if they
have little or no support. Many women embark on
parenthood with rosy ideals and little realism. Women
are thus particularly prone to stress symptoms as they
cope with their very varied situations.

Women also face major physical changes within
their bodies as they go through puberty, pregnancy,
childbirth, breast-feeding and the menopause. Their
feelings and emotions swing during their monthly
cycles as well as during these major life-events. Certainly men may suffer from 'mid-life crisis' as they
cope with the stresses of career or unemployment, of
adolescent children, then of children leaving home,
and their own retirement, but they do not have an
equivalent experience to the physical and emotional
events in women's lives.

Given all this it is perhaps surprising that more
special provision has not been made earlier in the
twentieth century for women's health, both preventive
and curative. Women have traditionally been expected
to work hard, fulfilling many roles, and their health,
or lack of it, has been seen as a part of their lot. The
political and medical fields have been predominantly
male, and women have had few advocates until more
recent years.

In the 1960s and 1970s women did begin to make
more demands in the UK for health care specifically
for them. Well woman clinics came into being. Support groups and societies exist for almost every prob-

lem and condition. Various telephone help-lines are available and 'phone-in' programmes on radio and television are ever popular. Women's health issues are aired on the media and in magazines and newspapers. Books offering self-help advice are available on many topics, and a wide range of non-prescription medicines are available, including homeopathic and other 'alternative' remedies.

THE WELL WOMAN CLINIC

It may be argued that the well woman clinic is based on the medical, the holistic or the self-help model.

The medical model emphasizes medically based prevention and cure, offering screening, advice and referral.

The holistic model embraces the woman's physical, social and emotional needs. There is a strong element of self-help.

The self-help model is based on support groups through which women explore health issues and a positive life-style. Health education is offered and women are helped to the position where they may make informed choices in health care and become more assertive.

Each model has its strengths and ideally elements of each should be seen in every clinic.

The well woman clinic may offer any or all of the following services.

General physical examination A medical history is taken; weight and blood pressure are checked; urinalysis for proteinuria and glycosuria is performed; blood tests for rubella status and anaemia screening are offered; the heart, chest and abdomen are examined. Cholesterol screening may be appropriate if the family history reveals a high incidence of cardiovascular problems. Other specialized screening such as sickle cell or thalassaemia tests may be offered in an at-risk population.

Cervical cytology   Cervical smears are offered. Cervical cytology is discussed in more detail in Chapter 29.

Pelvic examination   This is offered at the same time as the cervical smear. The doctor or nurse is looking for masses or tenderness. The cervix is visualized as the smear is taken, so that problems such as cervical erosion or polyps may be detected at the same time.

Breast examination   The breasts are checked by the nurse or doctor, and the woman is taught how and when to examine her breasts herself (See Chapter 32.)

The opportunity is readily available for the nurse to offer health education on matters such as weight reduction, stress management, the menopause, smoking, alcohol and a healthy life-style generally. The atmosphere and approach should be such that the woman feels able to ask advice on any problems or worries, such as psychosexual problems, vaginal discharge, child-care or contraception. The nurse should have leaflets available and should be able to refer women to the appropriate agency for more detailed help.

At the time of writing many changes are being introduced into general practice in the UK, and family doctors are being encouraged to offer much more preventive health care, advice and screening. Many women will still feel unable to talk in depth to their general practitioner, however, or they may prefer a slightly more anonymous environment. Many will seek out the option of seeing a female doctor which may not be possible at their local surgery or health centre.

PREGNANCY COUNSELLING

This may be something a woman seeks outside the general practitioner's surgery. A variety of societies exist to help women make informed choices about pregnancy. Some will tend to be anti-abortion and will aim to support the woman in continuing with her pregnancy.

FAMILY PLANNING CLINICS

A full range of contraceptive advice and services is offered. Counselling may be available on psychosexual problems. Cervical cytology is offered. The woman is referred to other agencies if necessary.

Some Family Planning Clinics offer the range of well woman services described earlier in this chapter.

Most general practitioners offer the full range of contraceptive services and advice, but the woman is free to choose where she wishes to go.

FURTHER READING

GOULD, D. (1990) *Nursing Care of Women*. Englewood Cliffs, NJ: Prentice-Hall.

MCPHERSON, A. & ANDERSON, A. (Eds.) (1983) *Women's Problems in General Practice*. Oxford University Press.

OAKLEY, A. (1972) *Sex, Gender and Society*. London: Maurice Temple Smith.

ORR, J. (Ed.) (1987) *Women's Health in the Community* (Topics in Community Health). John Wiley: Chichester.

WEBB, C. (Ed.) (1986) *Women's Health, Midwifery and Gynaecological Nursing* (Using Nursing Models Series). Sevenoaks: Hodder and Stoughton.

USEFUL ADDRESSES

Amarant Trust
80 Lambeth Road
London SE1 7PW
(Advice and support—menopause)

Association for Improvement in Maternity Services
(AIMS)
163 Liverpool Road
London N1 0RF

Association for Spina Bifida and Hydrocephalus
22 Upper Woburn Place
London WC1H 0EP

BACUP
121 Charterhouse Street
London EC1M 6AA
(Advice and counselling for cancer patients and
their families)

Caesarean Support Network
11 Duke Street
Astley
Lancs M29 7BG

Cleft Lip and Palate Association (CLAPA)
1 Eastwood Gardens
Kenton
Newcastle-Upon-Tyne

Compassionate Friends
6 Denmark Street
Bristol BS1 5DG
(For support following the loss of a child)

Down's Syndrome Association (DSA)
12–13 Clapham Common South Side
London SW4 7AA

Family Planning Association (FPA)
Margaret Pyke House
27–35 Mortimer Street
London W1N 7RJ

Foresight (the Association for the Promotion of Preconceptual Care)
The Old Vicarage
Church Lane
Witley
Godalming
Surrey GU8 5PN

Foundation for the Study of Infant Deaths
Fifth Floor
4 Grosvenor Place
London SW1X 7HD

Gingerbread
35 Wellington Street
London WC2E 7BN
(For single parents)

Health Education Authority
78 New Oxford Street
London WC1A 1AH

Hysterectomy Support Group
c/o Ann Webb
11 Henryson Road
London SE4 1HL

Mastectomy Association
15–19 Britten Street
London SW3 3TZ

National Childbirth Trust (NCT)
9 Queensborough Terrace
London W2 3TB

Pregnancy Advisory Service
13 Charlotte Street
London W1P 1HD

Stillbirths and Neonatal Death Society (SANDS)
Argyle House
29–31 Euston Road
London NW1 2SD

Terrence Higgins Trust
BM AIDS
London WC1N 3XX

Twins and Multiple Births Association (TAMBA)
54 Broad Lane
Hampton
Middlesex TW12 3BG

Women's Health Concern (WHC)
Ground Floor
17 Earls Terrace
London W8 6LP

GLOSSARY

Abortus: a dead or non-viable fetus born weighing less than 500 grams.

AFP: initials standing for alpha-fetoprotein. Measurement of levels of AFP are used in antenatal diagnosis of neural tube defects (a high level) or possible Down's syndrome (a low level).

AID: artificial insemination by donor semen.

AIDS: Acquired immune deficiency syndrome.

AIH: artificial insemination using the husband's semen.

Amenorrhoea: absence of the menstrual period.

Amniocentesis: sampling and examination of the amniotic fluid in early pregnancy. A diagnostic test for chromosomal abnormality.

Amnion: the inner of the two fetal membranes which surround the fetus, placenta and amniotic fluid.

Anteflexion: the forward bending of the top half of an organ; a term often used to describe the uterus.

Anteversion: a term describing the tipping forwards of an entire organ; the normal position of the non-pregnant uterus.

APH: antepartum haemorrhage; bleeding from the genital tract after the 28th week of pregnancy.

ARM: artificial rupture of the membranes.

ARM: Association of Radical Midwives.

Barr bodies: the sex chromatin which is found in normal female cells.

Carneous mole: a missed abortion in which the fetus remains *in utero* surrounded by clotted blood.

Cervical cerclage: a suture resembling a 'purse string' which is inserted around an incompetent cervix to maintain a pregnancy.

Chocolate cyst: a type of ovarian cyst.

Choriocarcinoma: a highly malignant condition arising from about 3% of hydatidiform moles.

Chorion: the outer of the two fetal membranes which surround the fetus, placenta and amniotic fluid.

Chromatin: the tissue within the chromosome which takes up basic dyes, allowing staining for microscopic examination.

CIN: cervical intraepithelial neoplasia (carcinoma of the uterine cervix).

Climacteric: the menopause.

Coitus interruptus: a method of contraception in which the man withdraws his penis before ejaculation.

Colporrhaphy: repair of the vaginal walls either after trauma, most commonly childbirth, or because of lax pelvic floor muscles.

Colposcopy: examination of the vagina and uterine cervix using a magnifying lens.

Conceptus: the entire products of conception at any stage following fertilization.

Corpus albicans: lit. 'white body'. The white tissue which replaces the regressing corpus luteum.

Corpus luteum: lit. 'yellow body'. A yellow mass which develops in the ovarian follicle after ovulation and rupture of that follicle. It has an endocrine function if pregnancy occurs.

CPD: cephalopelvic disproportion; the fetal head is too large to pass through the maternal pelvis.

CTG: cardiotocograph; an electronic recording in graph form of the fetal heart rate together with any uterine contractions.

Culdoscopy: endoscopic examination of the female pelvic organs via the posterior fornix; it is now largely superseded by laparoscopy.

CVS (CVB): chorionic villus sampling (chorionic villus

biopsy). Removal and examination of a piece of early placental tissue to detect chromosomal abnormality.

Cystocele: prolapse of the bladder into the vagina caused by laxity of the anterior vaginal wall.

D & C: dilatation (of the cervix) and curettage (of the uterine cavity).

DIC: disseminated intravascular coagulation.

Dysfunctional uterine bleeding: heavy periods or inter-menstrual bleeding for which no pathological cause is found.

Dyspareunia: pain experienced by a woman during sexual intercourse.

Dysplasia: abnormal development; a term often seen on cervical smear reports referring to abnormal cervical cells.

Ectopic pregnancy: implantation of the zygote outside the uterus, most commonly in the fallopian tube.

EDD (EDC): expected date of delivery (expected date of confinement).

Embryo: the developing organism from fertilization of the ovum until the end of the second month of intrauterine life.

Endometriosis: an abnormal growth of endometrial tissue outside the uterine cavity.

Endometrium: the lining of the uterus.

Erosion (cervical): an area of red, friable tissue around the external os caused by overgrowth of cells normally found in the cervical canal.

ERPC: evacuation of retained products of conception.

Fetus: the developing human being from the third month of intrauterine life until delivery.

FHH: fetal heart heard.

FHNH: fetal heart not heard.

FMF: fetal movements felt.

FMNF: fetal movements not felt.

FSH: follicle stimulating hormone.

Gamete: a sex cell; the sperm or the ovum.
Gender identity: the individual's concept of himself or herself as being male and masculine or female and feminine.
Genotype: the genetic characteristics of an individual.
GIFT: gamete intrafallopian transfer.
Graafian follicle: the ovarian follicle; the cystic structure housing an ovum.
Gravidity: a term describing the number of pregnancies a woman has had.

Habitual abortion: repeated spontaneous abortion; the term is usually used after a woman's third consecutive abortion.
Haematocolpos: a collection of blood within the vagina occurring at the menarche in a girl with an imperforate hymen.
HCG: human chorionic gonadotrophin; a hormone secreted in early pregnancy. Pregnancy tests are based on detection of HCG.
HPL: human placental lactogen.
HRT: hormone replacement therapy; usually refers to the giving of low doses of oestrogen and progesterone to postmenopausal women.
Hydatidiform mole: disordered development of the zygote resulting in a rapidly growing cystic mass.
Hymenotomy: surgical incision of an imperforate hymen.
Hysterosalpingogram: X-ray investigation of the uterus and fallopian tubes to detect tubal impatency.
Hysteroscopy: endoscopic examination of the uterine cavity.
Hysterotomy: surgical opening of the uterus.

Involution: term describing the return to normal size of the uterus following delivery.
IUCD: intrauterine contraceptive device.

IUD: intrauterine death.
IUGR: intrauterine growth retardation.
IVF: *in vitro* fertilization.

Laparoscopy: endoscopic examination of the female pelvic organs via the abdominal wall.
Leucoplakia (leukoplakia): development of white or greyish patches on the vulva; these may become malignant.
Leucorrhoea (leukorrhoea): non-pathological, white vaginal secretion.
LH: luteinizing hormone.
Libido: sexual desire.
LMP: last menstrual period.
Lochia: loss *per vaginam* following delivery; it originates from the placental site.
LSCS (LUSCS): lower segment caesarean section (lower uterine segment caesarean section).

Menarche: the onset of menstruation.
Menopause: the complete cessation of menstruation.
Menorrhagia: heavy menstrual loss.
Metrorrhagia: irregular uterine bleeding, independent of menstruation.
Missed abortion: the embryo or fetus dies but is not expelled by the uterus.
Mittelschmerz: pain caused by ovulation.
Multigravida: a woman who has had more than one pregnancy.
Multipara: a woman who has borne more than one viable child.
Myoma (fibromyoma): a benign uterine tumour; colloquially called a fibroid.
Myomectomy: surgical excision of a fibroid.
Myometrium: the muscular layer of the uterus.

Nidation: implantation of the zygote.

NND: neonatal death; death of the infant in the first 28 days.

Nullipara: a woman who has not borne a viable child.

OCP: the oral contraceptive pill.

Oligomenorrhoea: scanty menstruation.

Oocyte: the ovum before it becomes mature.

Oophorectomy: surgical excision of the ovary.

Oxytocic drug: a synthetic substance which stimulates uterine contractions.

Parous: descriptive term for the woman who has borne viable children.

Pelvic exenteration: surgical excision of all pelvic organs, usually for malignancy.

Perineorrhaphy: surgical repair of the perineum.

PID: pelvic inflammatory disease.

PMS (PMT): premenstrual syndrome (premenstrual tension).

PPH: postpartum haemorrhage; blood loss following delivery which exceeds 500 ml or causes deterioration in the woman's condition.

Procidentia: complete prolapse of the uterus into the vagina.

Pseudocyesis: 'phantom pregnancy'; an imagined pregnancy.

Puerperium: the six weeks following delivery, during which the body returns to its pre-pregnant state.

Rectocele: prolapse of the rectum into the vagina caused by laxity of the posterior vaginal wall.

Red degeneration: ischaemic change which may occur in a uterine fibroid during pregnancy; it often causes severe pain.

Retroflexion: the bending backwards of the top half of an organ.

Retroversion: the tilting backwards of an entire organ; a term often used to describe the position of the uterus.

Rhythm method (family planning): a natural method of contraception where intercourse is limited to the 'safe period' when ovulation is very unlikely. It is dependent on an awareness of the woman's individual menstrual cycle.

Salpingectomy: surgical excision of a fallopian tube.

SB: stillbirth.

Schiller's test: a staining technique used to detect potentially malignant cells at colposcopy.

Shirodkar suture: a particular type of cervical cerclage.

SIDS: sudden infant death syndrome; 'cot death'.

Spinnbarkeit: the type of mucus secreted by the cervix around ovulation; it forms a thready strand when stretched.

SRM (SROM): spontaneous rupture of the membranes.

STD: sexually transmitted disease.

STOP: suction termination of pregnancy.

Stress incontinence: involuntary leakage of urine when intra-abdominal pressure is raised, e.g. when coughing or laughing.

SVD: spontaneous vertex delivery.

TOP: termination of pregnancy.

Transsexualism: a condition in which an individual has an overwhelming desire to change anatomical sex; he or she feels more at home in the opposite gender.

Trimester: lit. third; usually refers to the first, second and third three months of pregnancy.

TSS: toxic shock syndrome.

Tubal pregnancy: ectopic pregnancy where implantation has occurred in the fallopian tube.

Vaginismus: spasm of the vagina which is so severe as to prevent digital or penile penetration.

Zygote: the organism resulting from fertilization of an ovum.

INDEX